STORMBORN

MEET THE WARRIORS WHO SURVIVED THE STORM
AND ARE DANCING IN THE RAIN

ELEONOR AMORA MARKLUND ALI LEVINE
ANN-LOOU TORELL CHARLOTTE DELPHI BJÖRNDOTTER
ELSA RAPUDI JESSIKA BJÖRHN KAJSA LEVANDER
KRISHA YOUNG LENA SVENSSON LIZA BUSTAD
LOTTA ASSARSDOTTER MARLENE MÅRTENS ASPGREN
MIRA HILARIA MÅRD NICOLETTE HALLADAY
SIERRA MELCHER SOPHIE BOWMAN
VIRGINIA SADA YORK YVONNE MUNDIH MBUUH

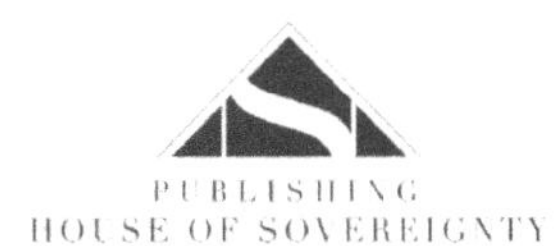

Published by: Publishing House of Sovereignty

Cover: MUSE

Photo: The authors' private unless otherwise stated

Print: Amazon, 2021

ISBN: 978-91-519-9209-9

To all the women who have understood

the true meaning of sistherhood.

Who do not back down when the storm comes.

To all those who have survived the storm,

even though they were broken by it.

We all dance in the rain

like the warriors we are.

CONTENTS

ABOUT THE PUBLISHER

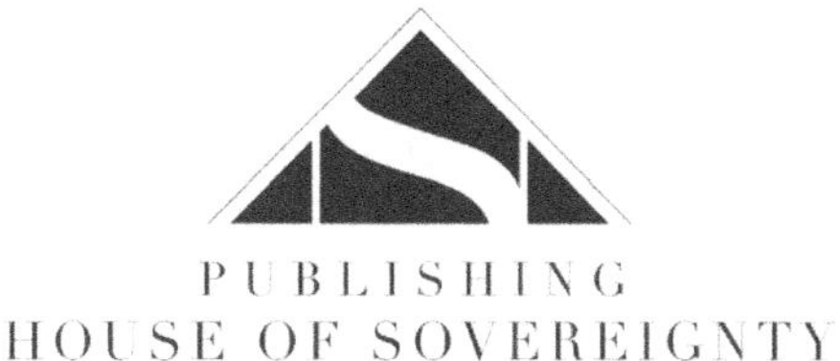

As leaders and influencers with a sovereign calling, we're driven to do our part to elevate the vibration of the entire planet. We know that it's our birthright to thrive in a reality of freedom in every aspect of our lives.

I created the House of Sovereignty to connect a global community of spiritual rebels who seek to own their power and achieve authentic, profound liberation in life.

The House of Sovereignty is a fortress that houses gifted individuals and strengthens their capacity for greatness. A multiplex enterprise, the House of Sovereignty contains multiple arms - from our sacred Temple of spiritual teachings and coaching, to our pioneering Tribe of free-thinkers and indigo warriors, to our media and publishing houses which helps spiritual entrepreneurs to own their voice and connect new readers more deeply with the Universe.

The House of Sovereignty is a global empire of pioneers that have chosen to forego the beaten path and step into their true authority. It doesn't matter whether you're taking your first step, or guiding others along the way. You're all welcome. It's a home for anyone looking to stand in their own frequency, master their abilities, and unlock their soul purpose, and be truly sovereign.

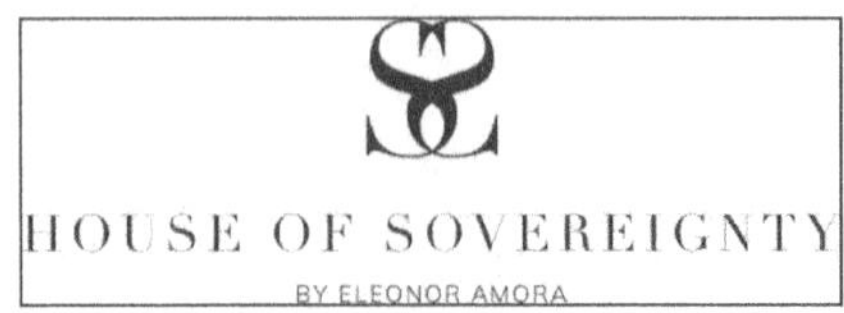

Many people dream of becoming an author... and with our help, this can become reality! The world's foremost spiritual publishing house, our team has created many best-sellers through our multi-author book format, but we don't just stop there.

As an award-winning, internationally acclaimed author with over 10 bestsellers, I also offer a private coaching program for authors that will support you through the entire journey - from writing and editing support, to design, marketing, and more.

Don't wait - start realising your dreams today! I am looking forward to hearing from you!

With love,
Eleonor Amora

www.houseofsovereignty.com

FOREWORD

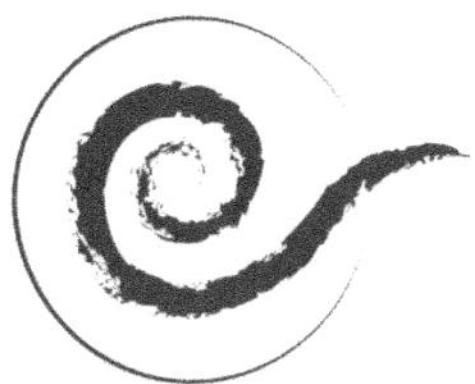

Sometimes, people who are interested in our book projects ask me what story to write... My answer is always the same: The story already exists in you. All you have to do is decide to write, and it will flow through you.

It is a deep knowing within me, that these books always choose their authors.

That as soon as you feel the calling, that is the tune you need to tap into.

Stormborn is not any different in that perspective, but what I love about this book is that each of the authors are telling you how it is possible to survive the strongest storms you can ever imagine. There is a stillness afterwards called life. They stayed true to themselves even though it seemed impossible at the moment. Their stories will tell you the tale of taming the storms in life and gaining power from them.

For me, they are the new leaders of the world we all share. They are forerunners, to show each and every one of us that we never have to endure anything anymore. We can raise ourselves and fly high on the winds instead of letting them push us down.

You have always heard your soul's calling. Even during the times when the feeling was only a small nudge, you have felt it.

I created this book project to inspire people just like you to do the sacred work that we came here to do, to embrace your sovereign power, be unafraid to use your voice, shape your own future, and allow yourself to receive the amazing abundance that is your birthright.

Remember - you can be your own storm and the one dancing in the rain.

With love,
Eleonor Amora

1

AWAKENING AND COMING HOME TO MYSELF

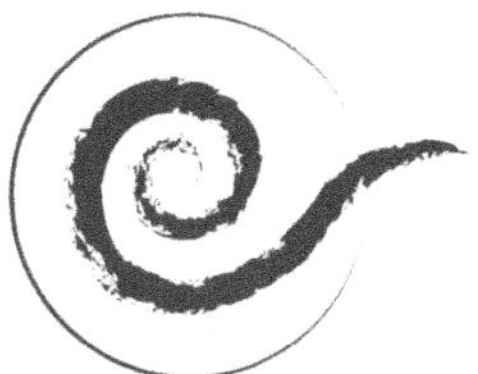

Have you ever felt like you lost yourself?

I certainly have and in that same loss, I birthed a new version of myself.

Being cracked open:

When I think about my awakening and what my soul has been teaching me, I truly get chills.

I've always been someone who lived on autopilot. Could never smell the roses in my life.

I would just keep going and going.

Going through the motions of life.

I would just go and go no matter what was happening, I always looked for the next big moment, the next high, the next push of my ego.

I couldn't be still or wanted to give myself time in a quiet space. I didn't realize it but living this way was actually making me be completely taken away from my soul and the essence and core of who

I was and am. The constant distractions and noise of everything around me, was keeping me away from myself. I felt like in those moments I was feeding myself (feeding my ego) and making myself happy, but it was actually quite the opposite.

I was just keeping myself from actually feeling.

I had been numb for so long.

The darkness that led to the light -

Dancing with the Darkness

My grandmother passed away in 2013 shortly after I got married. My world went from the brightest of days to the darkest of nights.

I could barely function when she physically left this earth. My grandmother was one of the most amazing and special women you'll ever meet.

She had a light about her that lit everyone up, she had an energy about her that you were instantly drawn into. My grandmother knew how to make everyone feel important and special no matter who you were. She was my true soulmate. It was as if our souls were attached.

When she passed, I felt my world crumble, my legs fell out from underneath me & I fell into a black hole. A black hole that just got deeper with time. I disconnected from my husband, my friends, my family and myself. I found myself looking for my worth in the external and giving all of myself to people that didn't matter at all.

They mattered to my ego. I stayed this way, totally asleep for quite some time. I gave and gave myself to everyone but myself. It was like a drug to me that I'd give myself and I'd get a mental high off of it. At the same time I was comfortably numb. I was going through the motions of life, I wasn't feeling, I was just doing.

Years later, I fed my ego with a reality TV show that I was asked to be a part of. Little did I know, I was about to go through a massive transformation and be shaken out of my numbness.

Finding myself all over again, Coming Home to Myself

I do believe God and the Universe will give us opportunities to grow and to learn and this TV project was it.

On the show I realized how much I had not been dealing with, how numb I really was and how disconnected I was from life and myself.

After the show, I felt I was shaken awake to see what I had been in and how I was just going through the motions. The blessing of this experience was not only being forced out of my numbness, but it also made me see just how dark I really was. It was like a huge flashlight had been put on me and I was seeing it all, clear as day.

Things hadn't been clear in years for me.

Shortly after filming, I got pregnant with my first daughter. It was the most magical and spiritual experience I've truly ever gotten so close to.

I knew my grandmother had picked her for me and it was all divine. I felt that energy from the minute she was created.

I had planned every detail of my daughter's birth down to every outfit for maternity photos, every detail of my "birth plan" and so much more. I planned on a water birth and a very Zen birth. The day to give birth to my daughter came and nothing went as "planned". I went into labor at home, went to my midwife and her birthing center and I was waiting to give birth for 30 hours. After quite sometime and realizing she wasn't wanting to come that way, we decided it was time for intervention and to go to the hospital. I was heartbroken and devastated. I wound up in a C- section after 42 hours and became bedridden for quite a bit of time. I could barely feed my daughter, bathe her, change her, I was failing before I even started this new journey.

The End of my old self and stepping into my new role and new self. It wasn't too long after being home as a new mom, that I started having very dark thoughts, and not being able to handle myself or motherhood. And there I was facing my darkness, my demons, it seemed like there was no light to be seen whatsoever.

I felt like I was mourning the death of myself and in that moment as I lost so much of who I was, I didn't realize I had actually been reborn.

Finding the Light and Healing

As I found the light at the end of the tunnel, and found my way back to myself, I came home.

I came home to myself, I not only found the light, it was shining bright and I was awakening.

I started seeing the darkness for what it was and working through it. Empowering myself to share the heaviness in my heart, the vulnerabilities within me that I never felt comfortable sharing at any point in my life, everything was pouring out of me.

I went from complete darkness to a bright shining light! I was healing myself and connecting with others along the way.

It was so cathartic. I never thought I'd get to the other side in those dark moments, but I did.

Not only did I get to the other side, I now know I had to go through all that heaviness to dance in that storm. I had to drown in my darkness to find the light. There's a beautiful duality when it comes to light and dark if you allow yourself to see it, feel it and move through it. You learn to dance with the darkness and not let it overcome you.

I now have not only come home to myself, but I am more me than I ever thought I could be.

It's almost like I'm relearning everything I ever was and forgot that I was and so much more.

It's truly magical and beautiful!!

My shift in consciousness has given me a sense of ultimate peace that I wouldn't trade for anything and no matter how heavy things can get at times, I always find the light and have that true inner peace. The more I come home to myself, to my truth, to all I am as a sovereign being, the more

I continue to raise the vibration and frequency for myself, for my loved ones and for humanity.

As I continue to evolve I uncover more and more in my universal search for authenticity, spiritual wholeness, and happiness. It's truly beautiful.

As I've awakened to much more of myself and my spirit, I continue to learn so much about the way I operate, getting to know myself and how I work through any darkness that enters on my path.

Learning how to journal out my feelings, words that were in my head and thoughts even if they weren't mine, being able to let go of them, transmute them and let them alchemize has been a constant practice. Learning to dance in my own darkness and find the beauty in light and dark, is something I come to learn and appreciate more and more.

What it teaches me about myself, how I continue to show up for myself, face the heaviness that comes in ebbs and flows and continue to flow with it and flourish from it.

Finding daily practices for me, and being honest with myself through the process.

Meditation has changed my life and my way of thinking. It has changed the way I process all emotions, situations and especially how I dial into myself. I believe it truly saved me when it comes to my postpartum depression and it helped me to rise above it all.

I also love breathwork, sound frequency, yoga, gratitude lists and journaling.

I think that when we can be 100 percent honest with ourselves and face our own demons and stare them in the eye directly, the more we find our own inner power and discover our truths.

That's how we ascend and shift our consciousness.

We are meant to live big full lives, super full. Our human journey should be full of learning, evolving, and shifting and in order for that to happen we have to keep allowing the process of shedding the old to bring in the new and allowing any part of us that we forgot, to re-emerge.

Soul Alignment—Everything I create in my reality is for my highest good and of alignment to Me

One of the things I've learned and continue to learn is being authentic with myself. If something isn't in alignment, I will not do it. Setting healthy boundaries for yourself and with others, helps us stay in alignment and be authentic to our truths.

Something I've learned over time, is that our truths are ours. Our truths are burning in our hearts, they are pushing and yearning to be spoken.

When we hide our truths, we only make ourselves smaller. Tapping into our truths, brings us into our sovereignty. It brings us back to our souls and our soul's purpose. Our divine alignment and what we maybe forgot that was always there.

ALI LEVINE

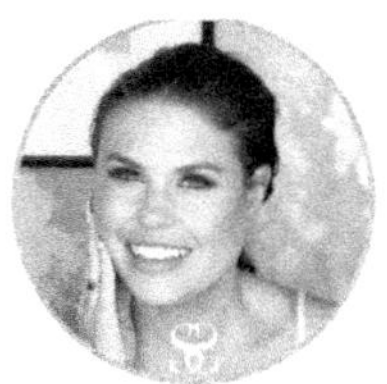

Celebrity stylist and motherhood/fashion/lifestyle expert Ali Levine believes that no matter where you roam, from the laundry room to the red carpet, authenticity is your superpower and "confidence is your best accessory."

After the arrival of her first child, daughter Amelia Rei, Levine wholeheartedly embraced the role of mompreneur/mommy influencer. She is now a mama of two and shares her real raw truth of motherhood. She is a sought-after motherhood style/lifestyle expert covered by *Forbes, The Wall Street Journal, NY Times,* and *LA Times,* with her work featured on national network television and in print/online media outlets such as *Real Simple, PopSugar,* and *FabFitFun.* She is also one of Yahoo's "Top Influencers to Watch and Follow in 2020." Ali loves to share her journey and what she's uncovered in the universal search for authenticity, spiritual wholeness, and happiness.

Contact information:
https://linktr.ee/alilevinedesign

2

WARRIOR OF LOVE

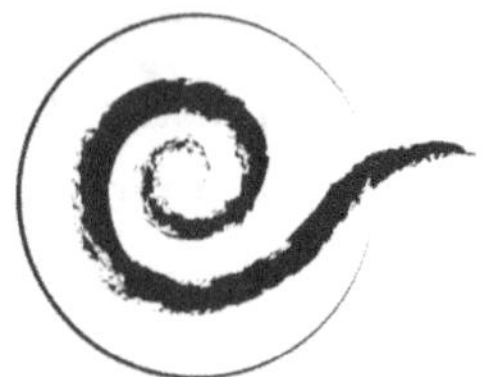

...When I close my eyes I can still hear her terrible scream, a scream on the phone that late summer evening in July. A phone call that made every cell in my body freeze to ice in a split second. Thousands of scenarios were playing out inside of me about what could have happened in those moments. This horrible scream drilled through every layer of calm within me, in a flash of a second I understood the seriousness and the panic grew like an avalanche, because I was not there and I did not know what had happened. I just hear my daughter Josefin's scream; heart-breaking and piercing.

“YOU HAVE TO COME AND GET ME!” she screamed, “He is coming for me.”

She continued with panic in her voice and it took me a while to get her to calm down enough for me to find out where she was and who was coming for her.

“Mom, I've been running into the woods, please pick me up because dad's going to hit me, mom it's dad!”

My whole body is shaking, I can't stop the tears and I say loudly, "I'm coming, I'm already on my way. Stay where you are." While speaking, I got off the couch where I had been laying dressed in pyjama trousers as it was already late. In my panic, I suddenly don't know where the car keys are but find them and both us, my husband Per and I, run out to the car. Instinctively, I felt that I should not go alone.

Earlier in the evening she had phoned me and said she was feeling homesick but after we had chatted for a while we decided that she was going to try for a little bit longer. After the phone call, it had been silent for several hours and I thought that surely everything was fine now, up until now I was in full panic mode inside and had to fight to not let my worry show in my voice. My two youngest girls, Josefin and Anna, hadn't seen their dad Allan for over six months. He had informed me that he no longer wanted to see them every other weekend with the explanation that "I ruined it for him." So it was better that they didn't come over at all. Once the children were older, they would come to understand what a horrible human I was, the root of all that was bad in his life.

In just a few seconds, I am in the car, still talking to Josefin on the phone. "Promise me mum that you won't stop talking to me, come, hurry. I've run out into the forest by dad's house," she continued to tell me. She was trying to get us to understand what had happened but as she kept hyperventilating, close to a proper anxiety attack, I began talking about what we had had for lunch at a café before I had dropped Josefin off and her 9 year old little sister Anna. Her voice was calmer now as we came closer. I just had to get across the bridge and a little bit further when I heard her once more scream loudly.

A man's voice in the phone, I hear it's her father Allan, then the call is disconnected. I feel how my foot automatically presses the gas pedal and I drive as fast as I can, just a few turns left and I say a silent prayer that all will be ok.

Once there, I see a small girl on the road, outside the house, with her small wheelie bag in front of her. "He" is standing with his arms crossed, leaning against one of the cars. Suddenly it all feels so unreal. Her scream was not long ago but at the same time I feel grateful that she is standing here, unharmed. I stop the car and we both get out. Simultaneously my daughter throws herself in my husband's arms. She clings to him with arms and legs like a little monkey...

Per is calm personified, not much can get him off balance or angry but I can see that he has to fight for it this time; her scream and fear hit him hard but now she is in his arms and he puts her in the car, quietly saying to Allan as he walks past him, "Good job mate" with a tone of resignation. I can understand that my husband is tired of Allan, he's had to take so much crap these years, that even he has had enough. Per's worry for Josefin as well as the million other incidents, made him finally speak to him. Then something goes wrong, as if the pressure has built and built in Allan, like a pressure cooker about to explode, you can almost see the testosterone in the air. A cockfight is inevitable. Allan, who couldn't bear to see his daughter seeking comfort with someone else, tries to push Per over, but he stands, immobile. Allan is pushed, once.. twice and falls over on his own property. Punches are exchanged, everything happens so incredibly quickly that I only have time to react and shout loudly, "Stop it, it's not worth it!"My husband Per lets go, goes back and the car. Josefin who is sitting in the car, has seen it all and begins to scream. So incredibly unnecessary I think as I offer my hand to Allan who is still on the ground. He gets up with my help, brushes himself off and it is only then that I realise that he is severely intoxicated, chewing tobacco is smeared on his face and he is upset, offended and very high on adrenaline. His huge ego has been crushed by a man he hates.

He begins to scream, "You bastard, how the hell dare you! I'm going to fucking show you!" as he begins to walk towards the car again. I know that if he gets there, this will end in utter disaster. I grab hold of both his arms, holding him tight as he wriggles and fights to get out of my hold, all the while spitting and hissing, saying how fucking stupid my husband is.

He says," I have cameras" and looks up towards the house where they are. I tighten my grip, try to get eye contact and say loud and clear, "I don't give a shit about your cameras, go inside, you're drunk. Think of Josefin. I need to take her home." I realise that I won't be able to keep hold of him and let go of him.

I walk towards their utility room, calling for his wife Karin, thinking that together we can stop more fighting, but as she comes out things just get worse. She pushes me and shouts, "Get off our property!" They both begin to walk towards our car, a united force, intent on creating more chaos. I have to hurry after them. I see how his wife opens the passenger door to talk to Josefin who is just shouting that she wants to go home. I ask them both to leave but as I utter the words Allan has already opened the car door to where my husband is sitting, his wife Karin has also gone over there. I quickly move over to create a barrier between them and Per, not letting him leave the car. Allan and his wife are after blood. They hit and punch to get to Per who is halfway out of the car and squeezed in by me so he can't defend himself, but at least they can't hit him hard. Suddenly I feel an intense pain, "he", Allan, has kicked me with all his might on my left thigh, I can feel that I wet myself.

I am in Allan's way and he wants me to move, hence the kick.

The next second all is still as if that was a signal.

From my pain the power grows and I scream:

"Move the hell back and let me go!". Both back up and into their house, like little vampires, afraid of the light.

Everything happens so incredibly quickly, the agony of my leg makes it hard to walk, my urine soaked pyjama trousers now cold and stiff, but I have to get us out of here and I don't want to show anyone that he has hurt me. Now, my daughter's safety and comfort is my priority.

But where is my youngest daughter, Anna? I make a last attempt to see if she is nearby before I get in the car to drive away.

The panic inside of me is immense, I have to get my Anna out of the house but I don't dare go back. The anxiety I felt when I had to leave, I knew that now all hell would break loose.

I start the car and something breaks inside my thigh. I swallow the pain, tears burn in my eyes and I can barely see the road ahead of me.

I hear Josefin cry, "I'm sorry, it wouldn't have happened if you didn't have to pick me up. Promise me I won't ever have to see him again, promise me mum!"

I answer her, "Sweet child, it's not your fault, nothing is your fault and it's a good thing that you phoned." My thoughts immediately go to my other girls, is this when I lose them?

I dropped off two little girls for a summer vacation and just a few hours later our whole life was like a war zone. Now we were all to be punished. The daughter we collected would be sacrificed, she was the black sheep of his wolf pack because she never let herself be controlled.

All us empaths became the losers, unlike the ruler of the darkness who got an outlet for all that had been brewing for such a long time.

He needed the chaos, the tears was what energised him. He is not like the others and in the near future we would all get to observe his masterful art of manipulation and lies.

From now on he would begin to gather his troops of "little soldiers" and these would walk united with a single purpose, to destroy those of us who were not on his side.

That evening was the end of so much and the following years would be an eternal struggle for us all, a struggle of survival and a deep sorrow that would grip all our hearts.

The coming years were hard to witness, to think so much evil can live in a single human, this evil, mixed with an incredibly skilful psychological game with only a single winner, “Him”.

Using all the tricks from the “devil” book, he succeeded in making three of our four children hate me once more, once more distance themselves from me, give me all the blame for this event and also distance themselves from all those by my side.

The tyrant ups the ante of the game, all those with feelings and empathy get deep scars in their souls that will take years to heal and to understand.

Let the game begin.

I want to ask you, as my reader, to take a deep breath. Close your eyes and try to disconnect your logical thinking and so, also your intellect, you must feel in your heart to understand even a fraction of what has happened behind closed doors during so many years.

When it comes to understanding a diseased mind, we go beyond our intellect and those with the gift of empathy, could never have done these things, that I will share a small part of, with you.

I will try to invite YOU to see through my eyes what has happened and is still happening for those still there, dancing his devil dance.

You must take a step back, see it all from a distance, try to see the unthinkable, that which is not easy to explain for you who have never been there and have never experienced it. Why do I want to tell you? Why can’t I just let go and move on?

Because it is still happening.

But, this was the climax. It was an era that had to be concluded for another to be born. I know this today.

I want to take you away from the shadows and into the light, I want to tell you that life isn’t always what we think it will be, that the sorrows and challenges become our lessons in life and when we choose to see them as such, it becomes easier to accept and forgive.

> "The hardest thing in life is to know which bridge to cross and which to burn."

This event was the breaking point of all those years of threats, lies and gaslighting. All those times when he sabotaged "my days" with the girls, making plans for trips and holidays on "my week" or the days when he returned the children and began to cry in the car telling them, "I have to leave you here because your mum says you can't stay with me."

So many lies, building their hate for me, painting himself as their saviour, rewarding them with material things so that they would understand that he was the right one for them.

That evening he chose to exploit what had happened by spreading lies, allowing someone else to take the blame. He played the perfect victim, he who never does or says anything wrong.

He decided to play carefully selected parts, voices removed, of the recorded event for all the children, young and old alike. He chose to use it to his advantage instead of telling them that things went wrong between two adults and that it was not anything for them to worry about. Instead he chose to take the opportunity to create chaos.

He needed more to soothe his wounded ego, he had met his match in my husband and now he felt threatened so he had to be destroyed together with everyone else who did not choose him. This was the time to reward loyalty generously.

After three weeks with the help of our solicitor, as I had custody of our two youngest girls, we brought her home. To begin with, we saw just small fragments of "our" little girl but as evening came, she was almost back to her usual self. Up to the point when she had spoken to her dad, Allan, on the phone and she came back to see me in the kitchen.

I will never forget what I saw, her eyes were dark, her small hands, who had just before been holding mine with such love, this was all forgotten now.

She looked at me and screamed, “I HATE YOU! I DON’T WANT TO LIVE WITH YOU. I WANT TO GO TO MY DAD AND YOU CAN’T STOP ME!”

At that moment I knew that I had lost her. She screamed that whole night, the same mantra over and over again, we couldn’t reach her, this little nine-year-old girl who loved us all and who had lived with us for six years.

She loved us all and enjoyed her life, now she was the one to be sacrificed. It was as if a demon had taken over her body, voice and heart.

A little girl was forced to turn away from those who were her family and over many coming years to listen to a ”story” that was not true. Every time she missed us she was served with the same lies, the opportunity to meet us was taken away from her, until all her memories of us were erased and forgotten...

SPIRITUAL AWAKENING

We have, in my belief, the ability to make different choices in life.

To stay in the shadow and listen to the voice of your ego, or to walk the way of the light.

To be a victim of all the bad that happens to us, or to make a choice of trying to heal ourselves, trying the best we can, to see that sometimes there is a deeper meaning behind it all. That the universe has a plan, sometimes it’s not what we want but we have to believe that it is for the best outcome for all of us, giving us lessons to learn, to awaken us.

This story is about Parental Alienation Syndrome, and that is in my world, an act of pure evil, not love.

I have been dealing with a tsunami of grief from the loss of my children and I was ill for a long time with post-traumatic stress syndrome.

But this is also a story of awakening, my spiritual journey.

To become a lightworker, I believe it was necessary to be so heartbroken that I felt as if I was dying, crawling through the deepest darkness. As if I needed to die from the old life, to be able to step into the new one. I had to make that choice of leaving the shadows and accepting that my life was not with all of my children as they were growing up.

I had to become the warrior of love and light so when my children have travelled their own journey in darkness, danced the last dance with the devil and are ready to step into the light, I will be there waiting for them, helping them to understand the deeper meaning, for all of us.

The ultimate test from the universe was to see if we dare to see all our own shadows, standing strong in the darkness and facing all our fears and in the end, be reunited in the name of love as lightworkers.

"Today, after six years of waiting my Anna is home"

I am Ann-Loou, Warrior of Love and Truth.

ANN-LOOU TORELL

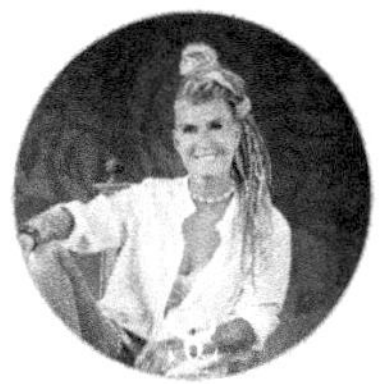

Ann-Loou Torell, is a Body & Mind and Soul therapist.

Honest, non-bullshit, spiritual life changing guide and bestselling author.

Ann-Loou has a home clinic in Sweden, but she also arranges weekends filled with yoga, meditation, fresh food and training for women both in Sweden and abroad.

Ann-Loou is well known for her powerful energy transformations treatments and also helps women face the difficulties in the golden age.

She also works with one-on-one coaching.

Ann-Loou focuses on women's empowerment. To help them become aware through knowledge and with that be able to strengthen their unshakable self-love.

Her life story is about her first marriage with a narcissist,10 years with psychological abuse and when she finally managed to leave, he made her life a living hell with Parental Alienation

Parental Alienation is an act of pure evil, but this is a story about hope, love and never giving up on your children.

Ann-Loou Torell

Website: annloou.com

annloou@annloou
Facebook: Ann-Loou torell
Instagram:@annloou_torell
Photo: Tallee Savage

3

BEING A LIGHTHOUSE IN THE STORM

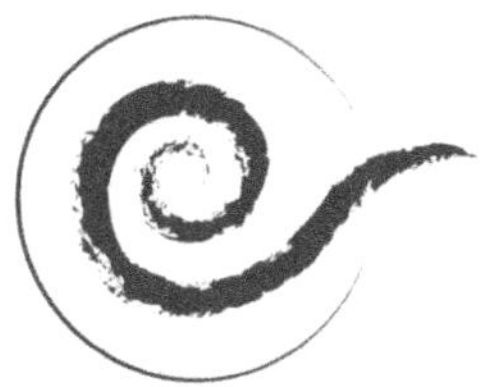

I stand in the middle of the storm
Watching the chaos around me
Feeling the despair, the sadness and the confusion
So many people and animals suffering
Nature suffering
Our sacred earth suffering

I stand in the middle of the storm
Watching the chaos around me
Shining my inner light, shining my love
Helping people and animals heal, opening up their hearts
Healing nature
Our sacred earth healing

I stand in the middle of the storm
Feeling unconditional love, compassion and unity consciousness
around me
Embodying my essence, being me, being free
People and animals celebrating life and sharing their love in unity
Celebrating nature

Our sacred earth thriving

STORMS OF THE PAST LEAVING WOUNDS

I have endured so many storms in my previous incarnations as a warrior of light but I have also been defeated by many storms. I have suffered immensely, being executed and killed numerous times because of my spiritual gifts and my psychic abilities. Being so different, being called a witch, being in trials, being rejected, being silenced and being an outcast. Living my life in fear, in hiding, being betrayed even by people close to me, not trusting anyone, feeling completely alone. Being a beacon of love and light, saving so many people and animals with my healing and psychic gifts. Being heartbroken over and over again when I ended up being killed for saving and healing people and animals. Not for my life understanding the logic in this. Being confused. All I wanted to do was to help! To make the world a better place. How can healing and saving someone be wrong? The worst was being forced to hide my gifts, trying not to use my gifts. Knowing I could save someone's life but not daring to was like torture. Learning to be silent. Learning to act "normal", to adapt, to fit in, to please. Dying inside. Defying my fears and accomplishing my healing mission got myself killed in so many lives. Condemning higher powers for giving me these gifts. Getting lost in all the drama and in the storms. Letting the storm tear me apart.

PICKING UP THE PIECES AND PUTTING THEM BACK TOGETHER AGAIN.

In this life I have had many challenges. I have been challenged to stand up and speak up for myself, to be brave enough to allow myself to use my gifts openly, to embrace my essence fully, to allow myself to shine my inner light bright and wide, to allow myself to be different, not worrying about adapting, fitting in, and pleasing anyone.

A FEAR OF AUTHORITIES

I have always had a huge and deep fear of authorities. It feels like this fear is ingrained in my body and in my brain so that I can't think clearly when I face an authority figure. My body fails me, my body language shows that I feel weak and submissive, I can't speak the words I want to say, it's physically impossible, and I feel so helpless and so frustrated. Saying yes when I mean no. Letting myself be controlled and subdued, betraying myself unwillingly.

A STORM OF FEELINGS AND ENERGIES

As I have worked with my personal and spiritual development since I was a young adult I eventually came to understand that, because of being an empath, feeling everyone's feelings and not being able to distinguish whether the feelings are my feelings or not, I had problems with knowing who I really was. I had difficulties making choices. I chose what the person closest to me chose, or what I felt other people wanted me to choose. Without knowing it, I absorbed other people's feelings and energies. I could feel so sad or confused all over sudden without having a reason for it and not knowing why. It was like being in a storm, being dragged here and there to extremes without any control. It was very difficult for me in school, feeling so many energies all the time in my energy system. Also, I wanted everyone to be happy and balanced so I unconsciously healed many children. I was so drained, so exhausted and so low in energy when I got home. I wanted peace and quiet and would sit in my mother's lap for a long time. When I grew up, my intuition got stronger as I acknowledged and developed my spiritual gifts. I started realizing that I was very sensitive. For example when I was going home in a taxi from the airport one day, having been in another city working, I sat in the back seat waiting for other passengers. Two men came and sat down beside me. I suddenly got so much pain in my back, it was hurting like knives. I was so confused. After about twenty minutes we stopped and the man sitting next to me left the taxi. When he was about three meters from the car my back suddenly stopped hurting. I understood that I had felt the man's back pain, not my own. I eventually learned to control my energy field which is very important. I advise everyone to clear their energy field regularly in the way that suits you best. There are so many different ways, using sage or other incense, essential oils, being in nature, surrounding yourself in a protective bubble of energy or simply ordering decisively unwanted energy to leave your energy field. Some years ago I felt a different energy in my energy field, a spirit, when going to sleep in a hotel room. I ordered the spirit to leave my energy field and return the next day.The spirit left and the next day I helped him to connect with his daughter who attended the same conference as me. It was a very heartwarming, emotional and loving reunion.

LETTING MY INNER LIGHT SHINE

Another big challenge for me in this life is letting my inner light shine, daring to be me, all of me. To use my gifts wholeheartedly and fully, without holding back. Realizing that it is finally safe for me to be myself. To be a lighthouse in the storm. I went on a seance many years ago and the psychic medium came up to me and started talking. "I feel a huge angel of light when I connect with you. The angel says that you have been a warrior of light in so many lifetimes. You have been stopped, you have been silenced, you have been killed. But you have to understand that in this life you cannot be stopped. You are immensely protected. Some people will try to discredit you but it will only be with words. Do not be afraid. You are standing in the frontline. You will heal and help so many people and animals. You will write books that are truly blessed by the angels. So be brave, be bold, be all that you are. The world needs you."

I have worked a lot with releasing fears and daring to offer my gifts openly and wholeheartedly. Releasing deep fears that really had a powerful grip on me, like being ridiculed, being rejected and being threatened, punished or even killed for using my gifts.

It hasn't been easy. Memories deeply engraved in my body and in my system warning me. "Don't use your gifts, don't you remember what happened?" But as I worked with these issues through my personal and spiritual development and aligned with my higher self and my essence the memories in my body and in my system healed and dissolved. I forgave all the people in my past lives who had hurt me and killed me. It was a powerful but crucial release. Now I could focus on my essence, on my mission, on shining my light. Being me! To proudly announce my gifts in public. "I am an animal communicator and a healer".

RELEASING AND BALANCING MY INNER POWER

The lion, for me, is a symbol for balanced inner power. The lion is the king of the savannah and is so majestic. Just by looking at the lion you can see and feel the lion's inner power, strength, confidence, courage and that the lion is his own leader. The lion just embodies these traits in a very balanced way. Therefore, the lion doesn't need to always show his power and strength, only when it is needed. This is true balanced inner power. It is all about energy and balance. To embody the energy of balanced inner power. Many people think that they have to be powerful in their expression in order to show their inner power and use aggression and dominance far too often. When I was practising to unleash my inner power, my inner lion, I was drawn to women who were very powerful in their expression and I learned a lot from them for which I am forever grateful. I learned to release layers and layers of suppressed power from previous lifetimes. It was so intense and so empowering, learning to speak my truth, standing my ground, saying no and creating healthy boundaries. But eventually I experienced that I started bringing the power more inwards, not needing to express it outwards that much any longer, instead balancing and embodying the energy of power. Balance is key. Yin and Yang. To use your inner power in a balanced way.

EVOLVING THROUGH DREAMS

I had a recurring dream from when I was a young girl. I dreamt that I was in school, in a big room with only one door. I was there with all of my classmates and a teacher. The teacher told us all to hide because she was going to let a giant lion into the room. Everyone panicked and started to search frantically for a good hiding spot but I just followed everyone, and everyone found a place to hide except for me. Then the teacher opened the door and the lion came, saw me and started chasing me. I always woke up right there in the dream, sweating in panic. I dreamt this dream from time to time for many years.

As I developed my spiritual gifts and worked with my personal development I came to understand what the dream was telling me. That I was afraid of authorities and that I was an empath, being the reason why I couldn't find a hiding place because I followed everyone else, and that I was afraid of my inner light and inner power.

When I understood all of this I worked a lot with myself and these challenges, making big progress as years went by.

One night the dream was back. Everything was as it used to be. But this time, as the teacher had ordered us to hide because she was going to let the lion in, I just stopped her. I went up to her and told her " You must understand that you can't do this to us, I don't care about your authority or your orders. I am going to leave now. Good bye". I went to the door, passed the lion bravely on my way out, looking firmly into the eyes of the lion and the lion looked back at me, giving me a big smile, and then I left. Boom! I woke up after this scene and I felt so relieved, so happy and so powerful. It was a defining moment in my life for sure. It felt like a graduation. I have never dreamt that dream again and I am sure I will never ever dream it again. Dreams are such powerful tools for personal and spiritual development. Cooperate with your higher self and your guides. Keep a dream journal, learn from your dreams and cooperate with your dreams.

LIFE TRAVELS IN SPIRALS

Our challenges, as I see as opportunities to change ourselves, to learn, transform and evolve come along in intervals during our life. Life travels in spirals. We face the same challenges/opportunities but in different situations and with different people. Life gives us lots of opportunities to overcome the challenges and it is up to us how we deal with these challenges. The first step is to be aware of and recognize the challenges that are recurring. Wait a minute, didn't I face this challenge in my previous relationship, and in the one before..? The second step is to figure out why this happens. Why do I react in this way? The third step is working on improving yourself and learning to react the way you would like to react. Life will then present you with opportunities to practise this. Every time you will get better and better at it and eventually when the opportunity occurs once again, it is only like a really small challenge, and finally you overcome the challenge, you "pass the test".

Like my example with the fear of authorities that was so deeply ingrained in me because of past life experiences. I have had lots of opportunities to overcome this challenge. As well as having worked a lot with my personal and spiritual development, I have also worked a lot with past life regressions and healing. My challenge didn't stop when my dream stopped, I have been challenged since then, but the challenge has decreased a lot. I experienced another great victory in my authority challenge last year. This time I felt like the roles were reversed, I spoke my truth with great conviction and without any fear whatsoever. I stood up for myself and felt like I had nothing to lose. I won a huge victory, and gained more respect and more abundance than I could ever have imagined. It feels like I have finally overcome this challenge as well as my other two challenges. For that I am so proud and so grateful.

WARRIORS OF THE EARTH

I am a warrior in this life as in so many previous ones. I am a warrior who stands firm in the middle of the storm, fully focused on my mission. A warrior is supposed to have weapons. My "weapons" are unconditional love, healing and compassion. I am a warrior fighting for an earth thriving in love, compassion, balance and unity. I am a warrior with the mission of building bridges between humans, nature and animals. I am not alone and I am not unique. There are so many beautiful warriors out there with the same mission who have also pursued this mission in life after life. I am deeply grateful for you all. Tribes of these dedicated warriors are now forming across the globe reunited once more to continue this mission.

Praising higher powers for giving me these gifts. Feeling the overwhelming love and compassion for humanity, for animals and nature. Feeling my essence, my eternal light, understanding I am an eternal being. Letting go of fears, there is nothing to fear. Letting my light shine stronger and stronger. Being the lighthouse in the storm.

Through the vicious storms ravaging the earth
I am building bridges of unconditional love and compassion
between humans, nature and animals
heart to heart and soul to soul
until all our hearts are united as one
beating as one
connected to mother earth
synchronizing with the heartbeat of mother earth
vibrating of unconditional love
and echoing into the universe...

CHARLOTTE "DELPHI" BJÖRNDOTTER

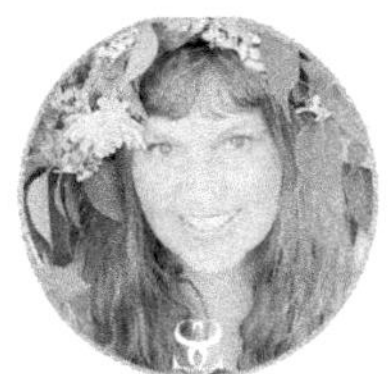

Charlotte “Delphi” Björndotter is a renowned, experienced and sought-after animal communicator and healer. Her mission is to build bridges between humans, animals and nature.To guide humans to discover a universal and divine heart connection with mother earth, animals and the universe. Opening up for unconditional love, compassion and unity consciousness.

She cooperates with highly advanced dolphin and whale spirit guides in the exclusive, powerful and popular healing modality that they have created together, called Delphi Healing. They also perform a very powerful “Star grid activation” healing session.

Charlotte channels the energy, wisdom and messages from nature and animals in singing and drumming ceremonies, guided meditations, swimming with wild dolphins and connecting with whales retreats worldwide, and animal communication and healing sessions.

She is a bestselling author with the multi-author book “Awakening - meet the women birthing a new earth” and a columnist in the magazine Inspire.

https://linktr.ee/charlottedelphi

4

PANIC ANXIETY - THE WIND MASTER

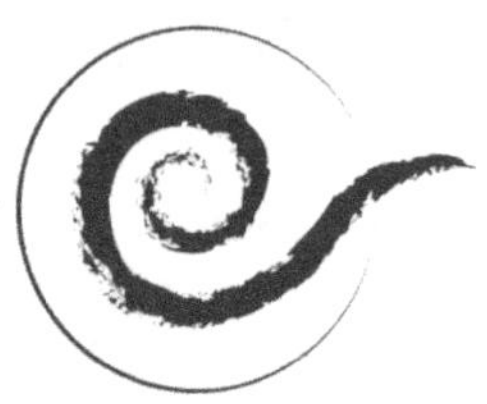

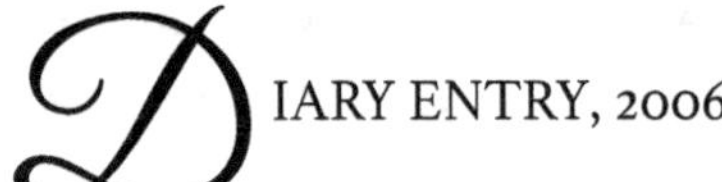

DIARY ENTRY, 2006

"How should I describe, be able to explain how it feels when the fear makes me incapable of being the person I really am.

A collection of emotions in my chest, where panic and anxiety threaten to break out, break down, break down.

The fear of nothing, everything, anything.

I can not breathe, do not think, do not talk, can not live. Not be a good mother.

I try to bite together, to stick together so that I can answer in short sentences and have a somewhat functional and accepted role as a mother. But I notice, he knows. He knows when to stay away from me. When I can not bear it.

When I can almost explode from nothing and everything. I have become the mother I have seen in my nightmares. The rage is not far away. Panic blinds and paralyzes. Why does no one understand? I throw something, anything, just to hear the cutting sound when it splits. Splits in the soul that never disappear. That's me.

Who am I? I'm not the same as I used to be and I do not know what I'm about to become. The fear of never getting well is reminded in every second, in every breath. I do not dare to look into myself anymore, do not dare to tell.

The fear that cuts through me that someone should understand how bad I am. How unsuccessful I have become. The panic that makes me unable to plan. Can not predict different events. Can not think ahead. Right now, everything is there and everything is. Just like an infant, I can only see the present and therefore meet the different needs as they come.

The fatigue that has crept into every fiber of my body. I fight it every day to get out of bed. To be able to care. It's not indifference, it's something else. Something I can not put my finger on.

The fear that gets stronger and stronger and that makes me no longer able to function functionally. No one knows. No one has the faintest idea. If anyone could see in my soul, they would be afraid of the dark. All the pain that I have to live with daily. I have no broken arm or anything else I can show. The pain sits in the soul, in the stomach like a great evil whirlwind; a whirlwind that threatens to grow into a tornado. I'm the windmill. She who stands there and somehow keeps the wind in check, so much so that it does not destroy everything in its world. So much so that it does not distort and engulf everything. But every day, the barren wind tears down my defense. The dams to the rivers of tears threaten to burst. Every minute I steel myself to maintain these walls and dams.

My soul is like a tense untuned violin string that can burst at any moment. Nobody understands that the smallest word, the smallest push can make everything fail. What then? What happens when the tornado engulfs everything in its path and sweeps away the little of the soul that is left.

What happens when I no longer exist."

A LIFETIME AGO

This year, it has been 16 years since I wrote those words.

I still remember my daily routine where I watched the everyday life of other people. It all felt as if I was watching them through a glass window.

I felt like a lightyear away. Like my soul had been dragged through the Multiverse and was just holding on to a thread to stay there and then in this body.

I had survived the abuse of my former husband. The fist. The rape. The narcissism.

If I had said or done anything that my husband disapproved of, he shut down the phone so that I couldn't call out, or shut down or changed the password of the internet connection.

From saying "I love you", "you can count on me" and "I will take care of you" when we got together, the sentences changed to "climb back under the rock you came from".

The memory of waking up, and realizing that all I wanted to do was get back to the sleep of no dreams is still vivid in my mind's eye.

One pill to be sleepy, and one pill to sleep the whole night.

I did what I could to survive. To escape from the relationship I was trapped in.

I had survived my suicide attempt, and I had returned from the dead. *(Read about it in Phoenix)*

One step at a time ... one foot in front of the other, I got away.

THE AFTER LIFE - OR THE LIFE AFTER DEATH

The first months after I managed to get away from my (former) husband, all I could do was sleep. It was as if the body had been so tense, so that I didn't even know how tired I had been.

At first, I couldn't distinguish between the whirlwind of anxiety, and my own being. It was as if the tornado was still there, in my stomach. I didn't know who I was any longer.

I thought the anxiety and myself was one and the same until then suddenly it hit me like a lightning bolt; I was not my feelings. The thinker inside my head was not the same thing as my feelings. The thoughts were something that I could start to control.

Every day, I worked non-stop with the thoughts in my head.

Whenever the repetitive thoughts and sentences from the abusive words I had heard day and night from my former husband started forming in my mind, I forced myself to end the thought.

I was like I was in a warzone 24/7, but the combat was inside my own mind. The thought pattern that I had lived with day and night, that repeated his words that I was not worthy of living.

WAS I GOING TO LET THE THOUGHTS CONTROL MY LIFE - OR WOULD I START CONTROLLING THEM?

Every thought needed to be actively ended. If it was hard to think positively right then and there, I chose the closest thing to think about that would be better, whether it was just a thought about the clothes I was wearing or the weather outside my window. Every thought was better than me repeating his words about me not being worthy to live, in my mind.

Every thought needed to be controlled:

> *Good thought - let it go.*
>
> *Bad thought - end it. Think about anything else but that. Pick something neutral.*

At times I thought I would never be able to succeed. The mishmash in my head of the years with a narcissist wanted to eat me alive. I felt like I was drowning many times. But still, I kept on doing it.

> *Good thought - let it go.*
>
> *Bad thought - end it. Think about anything else but that. Pick something neutral.*

Time and time again.

Day after day.

At first, all the negative energy that the anxiety had created had to be detoxed from my energy system and physical body, and this resulted in the worst nightmares I have ever dreamed in my life - before or later. The nightmares showed me death and destruction in every possible scenario, and all I could do was to let them take their turn.

Then suddenly one day, the nightmares stopped.

It was like the clouds lifted after a dark thunderstorm. The air was filled with the sweet nectar of the lush rain, where the energy and the sunbeams started to play in my life again.

From being stuck in the tornado, feeling like it would tear me apart and scatter my soul in every direction of the Multiverse, it was gone.

I had not known peace for many years, and the anxiety that once ruled my life was erased from my being.

I had managed to break the pattern of negative thoughts after living with a narcissist, and with that the negative emotions also cleared up.

There cannot be an emotion without a thought that precedes it.

And even though we feel that we cannot control our emotions - we can always control our thoughts. One thought at a time.

> *Finally, I was free.*
>
> *And finally, he was out of my head and out of my life in every sense of the word.*
>
> *The freedom to truly become the master of the wind itself.*
>
> *The freedom to truly be me.*

ELEONOR AMORA

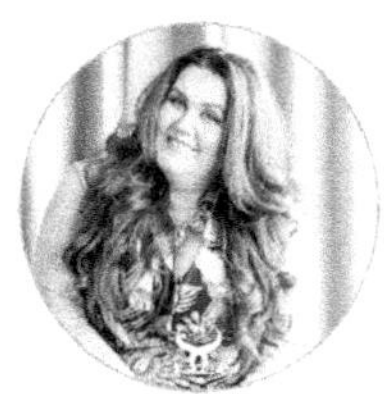

Eleonor Amora is the founder and CEO of the House of Sovereignty global enterprise and the Publishing House of Sovereignty.

An internationally acclaimed energy healer, spiritual coach and award winning multiple bestselling author who founded the world's biggest spiritual multiplex enterprise. She teaches everyone how past pain can be turned into fierce inner strength.

Are you ready to reach the stars?

Contact information and media: https://linktr.ee/eleonoramora

5

ELSA'S STORY

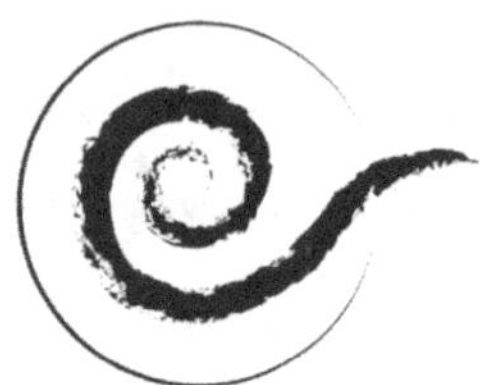

Are you following your dream life or living your life of fear?

I am talking to you from a place I lived far too long!

A place where I knew nothing about forgiveness!

My life was driven by fear and lack of courage.

It confirmed my belief that you meet people in life for a reason, like a fortunate strike of serendipity.

I am an eight year old girl.

Lying in my hospital bed, because my father did not want me as a child. He gave me food poison.

I ended up infested with tapeworm.

He sends me out to the streets at night to buy him beer thinking that he will get rid of me.

He hates me even the way he looks at me, I always feel scared whenever he is around me. One day he wanted to finish me off with an axe.

It was raining cats and dogs when he took an axe coming my way, I didn't think twice, I saw death coming and I smelled the end of my life.

I ran through the back door with no shoes on, no warm clothes. I had to save my life by running away. Lightning striked and I knew that God saved me. My dad turned back home.

I was saved by the lightning.

He ordered everyone at home that I had to eat my special food.

None of my siblings were allowed to eat with me.

If they did he would disown them.

It was hard for me, I sometimes felt like death would be the best solution for me.

I used to spend days without food because of his order.

I remember one day my Mom gave me food before his arrival and he found me eating.

He grabbed the food from me, went to our neighbors and gave the food to the animals.

I ran to the neighbor, hid there and when it was dark I ran back home searching for a secret place to hide.

I know how to sleep outside in the coal box.

I know how to spend days without food.

I know how to spend days without taking a bath.

I was terrified of such behavior.

The only place I felt safe was at the police station.

They knew me, always when I arrived there they asked me about my dad.

No one had any answers to what type of a person he was.

I remember one day asking the police to come and take him away from us.

I never wanted him to be prisoned, I only wanted him to be far away from us.

That's how bad it was.

I used to eat food that the prisoners ate and I used to be taken home by the police.

When my dad came back from our neighbors, he took all the pots and axed all of them. We were left with no pots, he said until we all do what he says life will continue to be tough on me.

I used to cry every day and night.

That affected my Mom so much.

When I was in the hospital, the doctors never thought I would see the sun for more than six months.I denied this deeply in my heart because I did not want to leave my mom suffering.

I promised her happiness, I wanted to see her smiling and living a normal life like other mothers.

I wanted to build her a house that she deserved and that always pushed me to work harder.

One day I asked my mom about my life. I wanted an answer from her, she kept saying "It will be ok girl, put your trust in God."

I started losing trust in my father.

I felt unhappy.

I asked myself these questions:

What wrong have I done to live like this?

How am I going to live like this?

I felt rejected.

I felt abused.

I felt unloved.

I asked myself, will I ever get out of this alive?

Again I asked myself how do I get myself out of this?

Is it worthy to live like this?

That was the moment I started to ask myself what kind of life do I want to live?

With whom do I want to live?

And I discovered that my father did not love himself and that's what made him hate me as a child.

I had no one to turn to, even my siblings started giving me an attitude like they weren't related to me.

No one came to visit me.

I decided to stand on my own.

I decided to love myself more.

I started to hate my father.

My relationship with my Mom got so strong to an extent that I did not feel safe without her.

I built a concrete wall with steel, not realizing that it was my own prison.

I trusted no one who came closer to me except for my Mother.

Anger, resentment and unforgiveness was my second name.

I did not know anything about forgiveness and I never thought I would forgive my father.

That went on for more than 20 years, living in hell. He told me that I am useless, worthless and will not amount to anything.That affected my Mom and she got sick with depression, in and out of the hospital.

I decided to work hard in school and in everything I did.

I knew that I deserved a better life.

And I decided to improve my life.

REFUSE TO GIVE UP

When things go wrong in life, when the road you're trudging seems to go uphill, go up that hill and take one step at a time.

Always remember that those hills are there to take you to a greater height for a purpose.

This reminds me of Margaret Thatcher who once said ,"I can be changed by what happens to me but I refuse to be reduced by it."

Do not focus your energy and time on things that will only remain momentarily.

Storm, my acronym for storm is something that only remain momentarily.

When life throws lemons at you, make lemon juice and kill covid.

When it throws stones at you, build a foundation for your own future and don't ask 'why me?'

If not you, who else?

Learn to breathe the pain towards its exit and know that storms are not always there to kill you, at times they are there to pave your way.

YOU ARE UNIQUE

Live full and die empty.

Build a legacy for yourself and family .

Most people are not living but they are existing in this world.

Make a remarkable change so that people will remember you when you leave this planet.

Don't be like those who don't discover themselves and aren't recognized at all, this is mostly for talented people with gifts inside of them.

Reclaim your power and pick up the pieces where you left them.

Because your story will be a beacon of hope for someone out there.

Your story will aspire to inspire even when you have expired, it will motivate and educate others.

So, don't mind all those who don't believe in you.

Impact and change the world.

We are all products of weapons of mass destruction, we are programmed to live a mediocre type of life from what God wanted for us.

Remember the price is already paid, we are not supposed to live in hovels, to dress in rugs and to live without money.

Stop comparing yourself to others because that will steal your joy, and comparison drives you only to see when you can't fit into your overflowing cup.

KEEP A POSITIVE MINDSET

Be grateful for your life .

Know that you are wonderfully and fearfully made.

Letting go of comparisons facilitates what you should be grateful for in your life.

Write your thoughts to stay on a healthy path.

Embrace the uniqueness of yourself.

No two people are the same.

We differ in our strengths and weaknesses.

Embrace your uniqueness of what makes you who you are.

Refuse to give up and commit to finding a way forward.

Approach the problem determined and motivated.

When you do that, it will help you develop a different perspective of problem solving.

This will create a mindset where you look at adversity as something to overcome and to solve, not something to be passively accepted.

Know that at times dilemmas and obstacles are there to create alternative paths, to dream bigger, push forward and even to take bigger leaps.

Be positive in every situation you find yourself in even how ugly it might seem to be.

Be your own shining star.

Speak life into existence about yourself and anyone else.

Never speak death into any situations or circumstances.

Have a purpose. When life gets tough, it helps to have a crystal clear idea of doing what you are doing.

Don't let your past circumstances refine you, let them define you.

Be a "no matter what type of a person" by following your dream.

If you have a purpose and a passion for your goals, you will persist until you succeed.

Be motivated and keep pushing through until you succeed and you become successfully successful.

Work on something meaningful for you, you'll always find a way back to it.

Do whatever you like, wherever you are with whatever you have.

Never give up in life.

YOUR ENVIRONMENT

Don't listen to naysayers and negative people when they don't believe in you.

You only get who you are in life, not what you want.

We all have one life to live and when you live it purposefully, once B is enough.

No one is promised to live a thousand years in the world.

Keep a positive mindset.

A healthy dose of optimism goes a long way when you are faced with a bad situation.

It may seem like a cliché but sometimes the darkest cloud has the silver lining.

Developing a positive mindset is an important coping skill when dealing with adversity.

It is true that you need to be realistic to see a situation clearly but should you frame it with negativity, you'll see only the bad side.

Cultivate positivity in every situation or circumstance.

Speak life into existence, refuse to let pessimistic voices and naysayers invade your mind.

Believe in your capabilities. People who rebound from adversities begin to believe they are capable of finding a way forward.

RESILIENCE

If you feel hopeless and powerless it is unlikely that you will find a way to be successful.

Have self-confidence and a strong belief in your capabilities that you will overcome difficult situations.

Believe in yourself and be open-minded and willing to leverage your talent.

Know-how and ingenuity to overcome adversity and believe in your dreams.

We have our birthrights that some of us don't know about .

It's up to all of us to claim what we are worth.

Adversity offers valuable insights.

. . .

Know that adversity is the best teacher and we all learn from university of hard knocks.

We learn from our adversities and have a better chance of success next time.

We learn from our adversities to become better versions of ourselves.

Adversities at times propel us in the right direction and they at times pave ways for us.

Embrace your adversities for they have made you the person you are today.

Rise up to the occasion and live like a champion.

Be a rise of Sharon to others and radiate love wherever you are.

Have eyes that see beauty out of each and every person you meet in life.

Have a mind that forgives the worst.

Take a hard look at your planning by considering your preparations.

Focus on an area that is within your control and ask yourself what more you can do next time .

Ask for help when in doubt, this will help you to become wiser and stronger.

I started reading books in school and making them my friends.

My marks at school improved.

My faith also increased.

I got my matrix results that favored me with university opportunities.

I was excited.

I showed my father my results, he never uttered a word. That also nearly killed me, increasing my hatred towards him.

My mom told me not to be too excited because there was no money to pay for my fees.

She told me “Why can’t you get a practical job?” I asked her what she meant!

She said I could get paid for cleaning floors and toilets for other people. I said but I am not ready for that.

It was my sister who helped me to think about training to become a nurse,

because I was not ready to clean floors and toilets like my mom suggested .

The college was too strict.

Firstly they were not impressed about my weight because I was chubby.

I was 2kg more than my ideal body weight.

They put me on their diet program.

Every month I had to check my weight before getting my salary.

It was hard for me to feel free like the others and to easily adapt to the new environment.

When life is pressing you down a bit, rest if you must but never quit.

Life is strange with its twists and turns, as everyone of us sometimes learn the hardest way.

And many give up when life gets too difficult.

Don’t give up though the pace seems slow- you may succeed with another blow.

I worked hard and I was among the five best students.

I decided to meet someone who could love me.

I needed a man who could live with me and take good care of me.

I met my husband.

The relationship was booming with good memories.

Years later, we were blessed with two beautiful kids.

Things were going well.

But one day, I never saw it coming, but it happened..

We started fighting for money.

I empowered myself with education.

I am someone interested in personal growth and leadership.

He asked me when I was going to stop educating myself because he thought it was a waste of money!

That was my aha moment.

I felt that I had made a big mistake to marry him.

There was no peace. I was told that I was useless and that I took money buying expensive books!

I felt that I had come to the end of the road.

One day we had a fight over my car, a week after I was hijacked with guns pointing at me.

I struggled to discover myself but I knew deep down that I would make it, I will be back on my feet again.

I was more into leadership and personal growth and he was not.

He was a ghetto man. My mom was my pillar of strength and I used to consult her when things were not too good.

During these crazy times of my life, my beloved brother died.

My two beloved sisters died.

I was hopeless and helpless.

I got divorced.

My God, I was now left with my kids and a huge responsibility.

I didn't know what to do and who to turn to.

God was my vindicator.

It's only Him who can turn a mess into a message,

turn a victim into a winner and I was victorious.

I have learned hard from the university of hard knocks but I never gave up on my dream life.

I tried MLM business but that did not turn out good, I had to learn to take a no many a times before I could become successful.

I joined another one of cosmetics, it did well but when covid hit the globe it slowed down.

I tried another one called PGI but I lost again.

One day as I was browsing on the internet, I saw Les Brown was looking for people to educate about how to use their voice.

I joined.

Finished the program.

One day I saw that Monique had a free five day challenge.

I jumped in.

I informed my friend Yvonne and she joined.

We even invested our money to embark on a 12 months program with her.

I was so sceptical, I never trusted to put my money with someone I didn't know.

I took a leap of faith and jumped in.

I started to become more visible on social media.

I was able to discover my story.

Was able to create a new story.

My life now started to change, it took a different direction.

I can now see the light at the end of the tunnel.

I can now sleep peacefully.

I walk in the light of God.

I walk in His strength.

I walk in His anointing.

CONCLUSION

Life is like a box of chocolates, you don't know what to expect.

No matter what happens in life, fight for what you are worth, otherwise all the things you don't want will take over.

Be grateful for your adversities; they are the ones that brought you where you are now.

Be grateful for your health, it's the only thing you have.

Be grateful for your challenges, they made you the person you are.

Be grateful for this beautiful day.

Be grateful for the air, the sunshine and the water and your ability to access them freely.

Be grateful for your body and the ability to power yourself through the day.

Be an overcomer in life in order to snatch the victory from the jaws of defeat.

Faith mixed with prayers and persistence can change any situation.

Never allow yourself to be surrounded by negativity and an environment full of drama.

Should that happen, pull yourself back and search for new environments..

Reclaim your life and evolve.

Live full and die empty.

Use your greatness and your gifts.

You are special, you've got enormous power in you.The same power that resurrected Jesus Christ from the grave.

I thank God for His Faithfulness.

ELSA RAPUDI

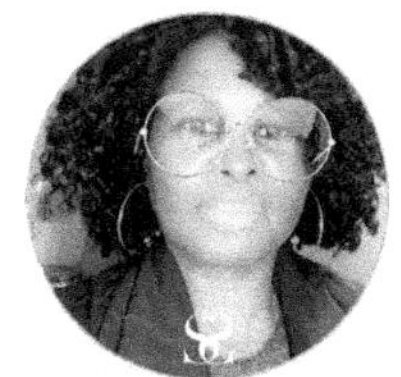

Elsa is on a mission to help others discover themselves.Trained as a nursing sister, she has 34 years in that field helping others to get well and face life again. She participates in African portal tv and in a radio station every Wednesday sharing different topics to the world.

She helps young generations and women to harness the power of their stories to make an impact and to touch millions of people.

She helps victims of abuse and rejections to forgive the perpetrator and to face life with ease.

She also helps women master the art of connection through the power of storytelling.

She transforms others by taking them through various stages, using her products to accept themselves and to know that they are greater than their circumstances.

www.pgsolution.org.

6

SHE BEHOLDS BEAR

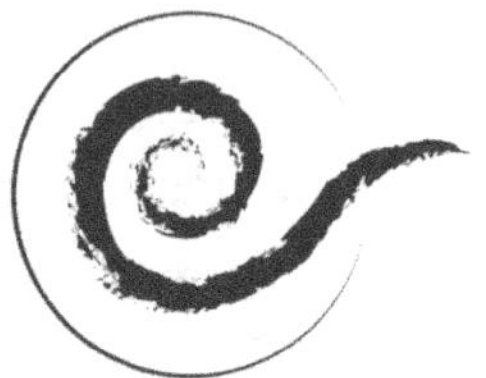

My lips were all blue, as if I had been eating blueberries. The umbilical cord twined two laps around my neck, like a scarf, just wrapped a little too hard. Something was holding me back. As if I regretted myself. As if I already knew that it wouldn't be easy. "*From the ashes into the fire.*" Just like Phoenix itself. I would die and rise again so many times that I had lost count many lives ago.

I was Stormborn.

My first encounter with Air in this life was not getting any. Not getting access to what gives life. What is the very essence of being able to breathe, to be, do and to live. Maybe that is why I'm having such a hard time trusting Air, breath, life, myself and others.

G-forces & Quantum leaps

As a child I would fall headlong into, what can be compared to, sleep paralysis. The creeping feeling snuck up on me as I knew that there was nothing I could do to avoid the inevitable - soon I would be seized by such a strong force that it made me tumble through space, universes and dimensions, at such senseless speed that I must have experienced g-forces. I was thrown down for what felt like an eternity before taking place in my body in bed.

As I started school it turned out that I wasn't able to inflate oblong balloons. My lungs and my diaphragm weren't strong enough. My best friend chose to start playing the flute and I chose the same as her. I sang in a choir and felt as if I had to sing as loud as possible just so that everyone else would dare to as well, since I have always been fascinated by the bold expression. My aunt has told me that she heard my voice through everyone else's celebrating Lucia in church, where I was close to fainting. Everyone turned their heads at me when we watched the recording from a musical in middle school. I didn't hear it myself but apparently I sang louder than everyone else altogether trying to act as support.

I would end up practising track and field. Sprinting and hurdling made my lungs reach their maximum capacity. I ran until air and energy ran out. My coach had to hold me upright so the gasping for breath shifted to hyperventilation and eventually normal breathing. The physician stated "Exertional Asthma" and gave me an inhaler. Looking back I would have stated "Panic Disorder" founded in deep trauma which was being triggered by pure exhaustion and I would have sent myself to trauma therapy asap.

I love running free. Barefoot. On grass. Crossing the small soccer field diagonally as fast as I can, taking giant quantum leaps. Walking the short sides just to gather strength to fly again.

Chasing Light

As a kid I used to play in the meadow by our house. I was chasing butterflies, talking to flowers and spirits. I climbed the pine tree waving a branch for the ones passing by. I wanted to amaze them. To remind them of magic. I often felt trapped but free in my own bubble. I told my dad that I wanted to live with indigenous people in the Amazon. Breathing fresh air. Living as wild and free as possible. One with nature. In symbiosis. One day there was a market with Native Americans at the big square in the small cobblestone town.

I was fascinated, didn't dare to talk to them but I told my dad about them. He, who's always busy, dropped everything to take me back to the market. All the way back to the indigenous people. He talked to the men, which I recall as Cherokee or Sioux. My dad recalls them as Navajo. Anyway, I asked for a symbol for freedom and I got it.

The White-Tailed Eagle

The one who doesn't fear heights or worry of falling. The one who trusts both air and its wings. It has a high vantage point and a sharp gaze seeing through it all, all the way to the horizon. Outside of bubbles. Passed small cobblestone towns. And far beyond the meadow behind our house.

By the age of twelve my aunt brought me to art university's exam exhibition. The very same year she also brought me to Stonehenge. It is told that every twelve years is a great transition.

Rite of Passage

A transition where we get in touch with our inner, higher calling. I wasn't aware until then that you're allowed to study to become an artist. That's when I decided that I want to dedicate my life to art. Ten years later I was accepted into art university, the first time that I applied, only twenty-two years old. The dream was fulfilled, just too early.

In my Bachelor exhibition at Konstfack I presented a fallen soap bubble made from glass, a massive sand castle so heavy it was hard to move and a rainbow projected in the air in a dark room. Outside the dark room there was a white floor with hamster cages and, what looked like, rigged rat traps. In the air above there was a cloud of bird cages which I called castles in the air. The installation had the title: *'Free Running - Too Fast To Leave Traces'*

Falling

After my exam I was working in a clothing store which eventually drove me straight into the wall. At a health fair I won the opportunity of practising military training. In February. In twenty degrees below zero Celsius we ran in deep snow. We did push-ups on bare ground and carried old iron bunks in rain and debris. I was the only colorful one having a hard time finding my running partner among all the black figures in the dark. After the last session 'Runner's High' turned into 'Runner's Low' and the last drop of energy ran out of me. I was done running. I was done.

At work I watched myself standing by the cash register packing clothes while lifting out of my body, looking down wondering what on earth I was doing. I went straight to my manager and said *"I'm going home now"* and that's what I did. By the beginning of 2012. The end of the Mayan calendar which was told to be the end of the world. At least it was the end of the Matrix to me.

It took me just as long to find myself as it had taken to lose myself being a working class heroine. I tried various kinds of healing. *Reconnective Healing*® was the reconnection with everything that I had repressed and shut down in order to act "normal" and fit into society.

I met my Indian "grandpa" who called me

Moon Princess

He read my hands, tarot cards and the stars. He gave healing, burnt his hands on my third eye, hit my muted Root Chakra with a stone, showed me the color flow behind my eyelids and told me that he saw a flying fish beside me.

The Flying Fish

The one who moves between water and air. Between emotions and psyche. Like a rollercoaster. Ups and downs. Ebb and flow. High and low.

Grandpa showed me the essential oils Rosemary and Lemon and the crystal Cat's Eye. I bought my first tarot and oracle decks with Art Nouveau and Astrology themes. Later on I found my way to the white lady's little esoteric shop where I didn't find what I was looking for so I asked the white lady who disappeared behind a curtain. As she came back she showed me *Shadowscapes Tarot* and I was amazed.

'Sacred Fire of the Heart'

During my Master's education in Fine Art I participated in Amazonian medicine plant ceremonies. I went from darkness to light, through all of the four elements. In my first ceremony I deeply regretted that I didn't set a specific intention. I had asked for everything. I spent that, almost unbearable, night in 'Child's Pose' *Balasana* with my hands shaping the mudra *Uttarabodhi* for the highest enlightenment. I had to remind myself to breathe. My own voice was calming me, reassuring that everything was going to be fine, that I would manage to go through all of the overwhelming downloads that flickered behind my eyelids. As I opened my eyes I saw half of the shaman's face as a skull. I knew that I was facing death. I rose up on my knees and in the blink of an eye all light went out. All black. Quiet. And still. All or nothing. I was all and nothing in no time. In the void. I remembered. I had chosen everything. Slowly the light returned. Or I returned into the light. I saw my small hands and feet as I was reborn into a yellow light and people cheering.

It was bright and I could choose when to dig down deep into darkness to retrieve information and to process things. All of a sudden I was hit by the insight that I had lost my mother. As if I just got the message that she had died. Now I was overwhelmed by grief bursting into tears crying desperately all night. I even wanted to follow her into the fire at one point. Someone told me I couldn't. Instead I was faced with another choice. Between a crystal ball and a black wooden turtle. Fast as lightning I grabbed the crystal ball. I still haven't managed to figure out exactly what it means but after that all went well. We faced the most beautiful and warming dawn that I have ever experienced. I had made a small altar out of all of my used tissues on the ground. It was a beautiful sight, small white clouds on the moss. As it was my turn to share I just opened my mouth not knowing what to say. What came out of me was untuned and fragile, I sang the known phrase;

"I will paint the whole world little mom"

I was wide awake. We listened to cheering songs performed by children from the Guarani tribe. My voice sounded like an old male tribe leader. A spider climbed out of my sleeping bag, which looked just like a gravestone and I found nails on the ground that I picked up. As I had asked for my purpose I experienced it as if I was pregnant giving birth, or not giving birth, I'm not sure. At least I'm sure it felt as if my chest would break in two as my heart opened in the last ceremony. That pain generated my only spit vomit which was thrown into the circle as I shot forward like a jaguar. I was next to the last one in the circle and noticed afterwards that the one in between me and the shaman had emptied himself the other way. We stated that the energies right behind the altar are strong.

I was initiated to share hapé and chose to participate in a Kambo ritual. I thought that I was ready to go through this cleansing right after grieving the loss of my mother. So I drank the required two litres of water as fast as possible and waited for the shaman who was away changing clothes. All of a sudden I got this feeling that I shouldn't be there, I sensed my mother's concern so I let her decide that time and walked away. On my way up to the house I met the shaman on his way back to the ritual.

The burn marks are traditionally made on the inside of the ankle on women. I struggled to pull my jeans up just to pull them down again as the shaman, seemingly surprised, took a good look on my hairy wild legs. The burns were made on my arm, just like a man.

The frog secretion is added and then you wait for a long half an hour of barely being able to breathe as your face and respiratory tract swells at the same time as you cascade vomit. I had to support my chest against a fallen tree trunk since it felt as if I would burst. So you throw up until you chuck up the little lump of bile which tells how sick you have been on a scale from transparent to black. My little golden lump was amber yellow. And it felt as if my body had died and re-emerged.

Water, Air, Fire and Earth

Every fourth ceremony you get a gift. Before the last one I was looking at the bracelets that the shaman sold. My gaze was immediately drawn to one with pink, purple and black pearls, but I thought it was too cute for me and found one with purple, blue and green pearls and a yellow eagle instead, but didn't buy any. Later on I saw the shaman grabbing a bunch of bracelets without looking, putting them in a bag and putting the bag in his pocket. There were four of us getting a bracelet. As the shaman came up to me he pulled a bracelet from the bag in his pocket, again without looking. It turned out to be the one with pink, purple and black pearls that he put on my wrist.

Later on as I considered going through more ceremonies than the four recommended, I found out that the shaman had passed. I was on an airplane on my way to a family reunion contemplating this matter when my friend told me. *"So, now you know."*, she said.

In one of the ceremonies I had noticed the shaman's necklace peeking from underneath his shirt, as if I was meant to see it. It was a ravenclaw holding a crystal ball. Afterwards I went to a festival where I found exactly the same kind of necklaces. During the festival I also experienced how a spider showed me another Peruvian necklace. A waning crescent moon made from bull's horn and a scarab flying towards the sun made from Turquoise. I met with a Sioux man wearing similar black feathers in his hair as me and we called each other brother and sister.

Crow Tribe

Our feet always know the way. They follow a trail. It's our choice how fast we want to go. To decide the pace.

As we were standing in long lines waiting to get in to the festival area I got this spell;

"Leopard-Otter-Owl"

Leopard for strength and camouflage on land, otter for flow and playfulness in water and owl with its sharp gaze spotting the way from the air.

All of a sudden the lines were dispelled, some people left and we were next to the entrance.

I held space for a drum ceremony singing the mantra:

"Jaya Shiva Shan-kara Bom Bom Hara Hara"

Jaya means 'victory'. *Shiva* means 'the good'. *Shankara* means 'the destroyer of obstacles' or 'the destroyer of doubt'. *Bom* means 'praise' and *Hara* means 'the one who removes harm'. *"Victory to the good, the destroyer of all obstacles and doubt, praise the one removing harm"*

We reached some kind of rapture where we burnt our underwear and walked on embers. I thought that my feet would be burned. Surprisingly they were just a bit sooty and it didn't hurt at all. No wonder. I started to lose balance and had a hard time finding my way back to the ground, back to here and now. It's easy getting lost in the magic realm, mixing things up in between timelines and dimensions before you've found enough support and tools to stay grounded. I'm forever grateful for some shaman friends coming to my rescue, taking me to a workshop in Norse Sha(wo)manism at a very special healing place in the care of an amazing Shawoman.

I got in touch with my everyday sha(wo)manism, guiding me to remove some really scary books from a book shelf. Showing me how my own limiting words and beliefs are affecting my work. At one point I was standing in front of a mirror, watching my face getting covered by a grey veil until my self-love shone through making the veil disappear. As I told the Shawoman she seemed both terrified and relieved at the same time as she hugged me and cheered *"You made it!"*

I was introduced to the tradition of '*Sejd*' where I heard my own voice transform from a masculine tone into a more feminine one. I got a rattle made from seed capsules, Lodolite dream stones and a Labradorite Ema-egg with a natural pentagram in it. I was introduced to runes and experienced several powerful drum journeys where I realised how I work with the four elements and met two power animals. My family name means bear and I have met the wolf myself in a guided meditation. Growing up with three German Shepherds it makes total sense.

During one of the drum journeys I was alone on an empty beach at a deserted island and I watched the ocean split in two. A pegasus came running in the middle of the ocean to take me away. On another journey, I saw me and my partner's ceremony. I created this stunning, lush elf-like landscape where we all gathered. It started to burn and I called in the rain. To protect us against the rain I had a soap bubble blown all around the gathering. In the underworld everything had turned into gold, due to too much alchemy, so someone else had to refill my fountain with water. In the upper world I was sitting on a cloud surrounded by so many flying dragons that I had a hard time believing what I actually saw. One of the dragons came up beside me, but I hesitated. Until the dragon hit me with its tail, inviting me to climb up so that we could take off.

JESSIKA BJÖRHN

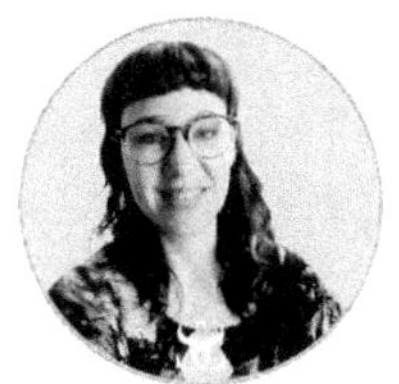

Jessika Björhn is a professional artist holding a Master's Degree in Fine Art from Umeå Art Academy and a Bachelor's Degree from Konstfack - University College of Arts, Crafts and Design in Stockholm, Sweden. Writing her Master Essay she gave a lecture on intuition, trusting your process, following the white rabbit and finding the golden thread.

Jessika has deepened her perspective beyond the physical into divination through practicing shamanism and by participating in Amazonian 'Sacred Fire of the Heart' ceremonies. She is inspired by witchcraft, alchemy, feminism, herstory, ecology, psychology, philosophy and spirituality.

Jessika teaches blind drawing, cut-up poetry, staged photography, left-hand croquis, tarot, sha(wo)manism and curates exhibitions. She has been published in various exhibition catalogs, anniversary books and web-based art magazines. In 2018 she participated in the 12th Shanghai Biennale. Since then she is also represented at ICIA - Institute of Contemporary Ideas & Art.

www.linktr.ee/shebeholds

7

THE WAY OF THE SPIDERWOMAN

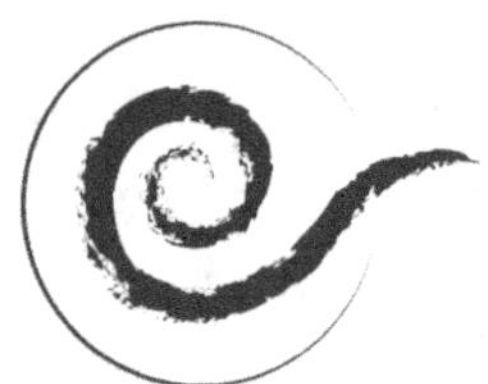

As an engineer working with indoor air quality and climate, I tend to get a bit formal in my written language. Although my most important tool is listening, connecting and building trust with the people who suffer from spending time in an unhealthy building. That requires authenticity and looking at the problem from a holistic point of view, not only from the technical point of view. That's where Heart 2 Heart communication comes in. This is about the communication between hearts and not a technical report. So, the Spiderwoman has assisted me with this text.

The Spiderwoman is an old shamanic woman that shows herself in many different forms. One of her signums is her very big drum with a colorful spider web painted on it and spiders in many forms. She is very loving and sharp as a whip. Just like the spider that is using its net for hatching and catching its prey.

The core of her teachings is balance and to stay connected to both mother earth and the spirit realm. In order to do that weave your web of life (of history and energy,) wisely. Strong and flexible enough to hold you when The Storm is roaring around you. The construction is important to keep you safe and on your path of life. Listen to your heart and live your life according to that.

Often when we find ourselves in the middle of a storm it is easy to feel hopeless and overwhelmed. But remember that life does not want to harm you. With your feet rooted in the ground and a strong web in your heart and mind you can ride out any storm and come out stronger and wiser.

Happiness and love is a mindset, not something that's happening to you. If you listen to your heart with a happy and loving mindset you will find your way to balance on the sometimes narrow and steep path in the storm.

Living is a constant work far from just passing through life and just letting it hit you like a leaf blowing in the wind. You are accountable for the way you chose to live your life, it's your choice, no one else's!

Everything needs balance so you need the connection to your roots and to mother earth as well as the spirit realm. You need to remember that you are living here and now in this linear time. Everything in life needs balance to be well, the light needs the dark, yin and yang and so on. This means that you need to be in contact with all aspects of you, not only the parts you like. If you really listen to your heart, you will find your own path to balance. Weave your web wisely so that it will hold you when it needs to. Strong and flexible enough to bounce you out in the unknown when you need to embrace the magical transformation from scared to excited. One baby step at a time. As long as you move forward, it doesn't matter how long your strides are, you are getting there.

I know that it can be rather frustrating when you are stuck in the mud. But maybe you are stuck because you are supposed to find your balance first. Take a deep relaxing breath and look for the diamonds in the mud. They are there, however small they may seem. Look at the sparkling diamonds and what they will tell you, that's how to find the way forward in a sticky situation.

The path towards your magical life sometimes feels effortless and sometimes like the seventh circle of hell. As long as you listen to your true self you will get there. It's always communication between hearts that's the key. But first, you need to have a strong communication with your own heart.

When you live your life accordingly your tribe or pack will probably change. You will lose some that cannot stand that you are stepping into your true self and gain some that are corresponding with your vibration. That can be a difficult part of your transformation, but you can't live your magical life by focusing on how to please others. It simply is not possible. Another important step is that you need to forgive and release that burden of wrongdoings towards yourself and others. This does not mean that you don't need to take responsibility for your actions. Nor does it mean that you are letting it happen again. But you won't carry the burden of holding a grudge. It's all for your own sake of mind. Release it to the universe and live your life with focus on what's serving you. Do not focus on what wrongdoings have been done to you. The power of accepting things that you can't change is huge and makes your vibration more harmonic. The need for explaining and defending yourself disappears.

Listen to the animals, they are generally particularly good at living here and now. But of course, they are also affected by their history and energy. So, treat them with respect and love, they will do the same to you, according to their own reality. A poisonous snake is a hunter that uses its venom to kill its prey and protect itself. So don't expect it to be all cuddly with you. You need to use your heart and brain to behave properly towards all individuals. The balance between the heart and the brain is important to all communication.

When you need to enforce boundaries, which sometimes is important in all relationships, be sure to do that from your heart and with good intentions. Occasionally that means that you need to use the force of your anger to make the message clear enough. Then it's even more important that you have put a lot in the "relationship-account" if you want to keep that relationship. When you use anger, you create distance. You cannot create balanced relationships based on distance and fear.

When you meet anger from another individual you have a choice how to react. Meet it with your own anger, calmly stand your ground, back off or just ignore it.

The way of the spider woman can be condensed down to balance. It is simple but not easy. Everything else is how to create that balance. How to find your path and how to stay on it. More often than not, it takes a few storms to find your true strength. So that you can navigate on your own path no matter what.

You can't compare your storms to anybody else's because they are yours. Depending on how you choose to live your life your actions create reactions. The history, energy and actions as well as your vibration is how your web is woven. Weave your web like the spider, strong enough to withstand the challenges life throws at you but stretchy enough to bend without breaking when your path is bending around a corner. Weave it with balance in mind. Let it be beautiful and magical. It's about how to fight sometimes with brutal force and strength. But often with wisdom, intelligence and love. When fighting fire with fire or fighting fire with love you are getting two very different battles. That means that you need to know when to choose what kind of weapon. Heat is melting ice, but water is stoking the fire.

Balance means that you need to find out when to stay firm in your heart and let your brain follow. And when to let the brain lead without missing the messages from your heart and intuition. To be balanced you need all aspects of you and use them wisely. The heart is the key to that information.

You have your beautiful web of strings that you need to weave together in all its colorful glory. All the threads are equally important but not equally strong and that's fine. You cannot jump between them and definitely not weave a few at a time. Trust your strength and ability. You have everything that you need, you need to let your magic sparkle!

Stay in your energy, don't let it leak to others. Just let your vibration be balanced and stay that way, into your true self. It's time to step up your game and take responsibility for your own path. Stop focusing on where you got stuck in the mud. Just let it go, otherwise you will stay there in the mud. Your life might not have been an easy one, but the rest of it must not be so hard either. Remember that happiness and love is a conscious state of mind.

The transformative journey from the brain to the heart and the communication between hearts is a really powerful one. When you use your heart's intelligence in communication it does not matter if you are communicating with humans or other species. You do it with love and respect. A love that's without demands and expectations but not without boundaries.

If you want to work with a horse, set up the exercise for success and reward (with something the horse wants) the movements in the right direction. Try to not apply pressure and reward with letting the pressure go. Even a small horse is big, and we have to think about safety too. So set up the exercise to minimize the risk for both trainer and animal. Be present in your heart and read the body language and other signals that the horse gives us, in order to establish communication with that animal. That means that you sometimes need to create boundaries, for example be on different sides of the fence in the beginning.

The same applies if you are communicating with humans. You communicate from an authentic heart but you have your boundaries. Heart 2 Heart communication is not about letting the whole world into your energy field. Quite the opposite, It's almost a ceremonial way of communication where you stand strong in your vibration and energy field and connect to the other individual through an energy thread between your hearts. I stand in my energy field, and you stand in yours. We meet each other with our hearts in the space between us. That means that we can have a loving communication, but we don't mix the energies. It's like we open a window and communicate through it, but we still hold our own space.

Weave your web of life wisely. Strong and flexible enough to hold you when the storm hits.

Build the balance through conscious weaving of your life threads to stand strong and connected in the center of the web. Get back to the roots and let the core of your soul be nurtured by mother nature. Go outside and let the heart show you what you need to be safe and grounded. Use the wisdom of those who have wandered here before. You have the knowledge from your ancestors within you. You only have to listen. Go out and connect with that old fir tree or that delicate little flower, they will tell you what you need. Put your seeds in the ground and see that they have the right amount of water and sunshine in the perfect soil to be able to grow. Find your balance between action and relaxation.

Listen to the wind, it's not always roaring, sometimes it's just whispering. Use your senses to find how to navigate in the wind. When to walk into the calm spot in the center of the storm, when to stand your ground and ride it out and when to spread your wings and soar up in the sky. All senses are equally important even if some are stronger than others. Strengthen the strong ones and train the others and always listen to your heart. Even if the message seems scary and not logical at all, the heart always knows.

Let the rain clear your mind and make you stand strong and balanced. Let the sun warm your heart and make you dance even in cold winter snow. When overwhelmed, use your breath to connect with your heart again. As you are focusing on that slow deep breath the brain can't do much else and it gets much easier to hear the song of the heart. Listen to it and dance with it. Let your heart lead you in the dance of your inner fire. Nurture that fire and trust it to keep you warm and moving forward on your path. Light a fire, it might be a small candle or a big log fire out in the woods, but light it and connect to the fire in your heart. Look around you and acknowledge the fire in the hearts around you. Embrace it and spread a wildfire of joy and dancing hearts.

Go out and look at the storming ocean and feel the power and the strength of the waves. Roll with them, don't fight them, accept their force and let them carry you from one place to another. Let the storming waves work for you, not against you.

If you on the other hand feel that you're wandering in a desert and all the water you can see is frozen, you're not just feeling enough, you're not needing enough. You can melt it if you want to use your fire and your determination. Because you need to melt it so you can drink and survive. In other words, you are not your feelings, but you have to feel your feelings. If you just try to ignore them they would get stuck in your system and that's no way to live. If you really acknowledge them and stand in the feeling, then they can pass through your system. Or you can benefit from the feeling. Otherwise, there is a huge risk that the feelings get stuck and feel like frozen water in the desert.

Let your pain be a guide to your path and not an excuse to wander off. Let it be a source for your strength and a pointer in the right direction. If you let your pain derail you from your path then you easily get stuck between the threads, like the spider's prey. When the pain makes you lose direction, tap into that feeling and find out what the gift of the situation is. Focus on that and the magic in a bad or hurtful situation will reveal itself. Realize that your vulnerability is also one of your core strengths. When you realize and learn to love yourself then you can change or insert them into your conscious personality as well as your heart.

Get centered and feel your power, the power of love. Let it flow through you to benefit both you and your surroundings. Listen to your heart and let your vibration heal your body and soul. When you're letting the loving vibration flow freely in your system, the pain melts away and the strength becomes more visible. Sometimes the modern world doesn't allow you to follow your ideal rhythm, then you need to create conscious timeframes to balance your vibration and phase, in order to stay in balance.

It's all about the choices you make. You always have a choice! If you stop and listen to your heart and not the brain or the gut your choices get much clearer. Some choices you have to repeat every day and some you just change, and then it's done. It's allowed to change one's mind but it's better to do that consciously and not like a leaf blowing in the wind. Stay focused on your vibration to shield you from letting other energies in.

We always come back to the fact that your heart knows your path, so make the effort to learn to listen to your heart. At least do that connection the first thing in the morning and the last thing at night. Listen to the huge wisdom of your heart. It's easy to just take a conscious breath and just listen in. Then you need to use your beautiful brain to carry out your heart's instructions. Stay focused on your core vibration to shield you from leaking energies or letting the wrong things in. Use whatever tool you need to stay focused; it might be a drum, some scents or your breath. Find out what's helping you and use it every day. In order to really be there for another being you have to be there for yourself.

Love people enough to not save them from themselves time after time. The loving thing is sometimes to do nothing at all. You can't do the journey for someone else, because they won't learn. What you can do is be there and support them while they are doing it by themselves. Everybody has to weave their own web, it's simply impossible to do it for somebody else. Not even for your children. If you try, there is a risk that they fall in between the threads. Be a loving and supporting guide for your surroundings, but do not try to do it for them.

Acknowledge your fears and let go of what's not serving you anymore. Leave it to mother earth and the universe to take care of. You get what you are sending out, so as long as the lesson isn't learned, it will come in return.

If you want to find your balance you need to follow your personal route, with love and trust for the journey ahead. But you also have to do your work. With a strong bond to mother nature, her gifts and cycles, but also to have an understanding for the spirit realm as well as the here and now. Don't forget that magic is manifestations in action. And it's happening everywhere. Go out and create your magical life! You have got everything you need within you, use it well!

KAJSA LEVANDER

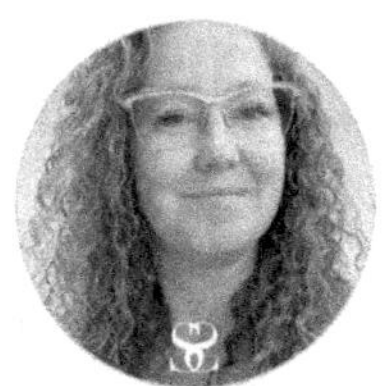

Kajsa is a versatile entrepreneur, engineer, bestselling author and inspirator who coaches people and animals.

Kajsa is CEO of Byggnadsmiljö Mellansverige AB, which includes Quartet Dog Training and Quartet Coaching. Health is close to her heart, whether it's buildings, people, animals or nature.

As an animal trainer, Kajsa is driven by the collaboration with the animals based on their choice to collaborate. This has led Kajsa to develop her special interests, behavioral analysis and scent detection.

With a background as a dog trainer and coach, she has developed Heart 2 Heart Communication, to incorporate people and their well-being with a responsiveness to the animals.

Kajsa's work to support people and animals means that she incorporates old wisdom from previous generations into our time. Among other things, meditation, relaxation techniques, essential oils from doTERRA and Shamanic methods in harmony with Mother Pinetree's Wisdom®.

https://linktr.ee/Kvartett

8

THE VICTIM MENTALITY AND HOW IT SAVED MY LIFE

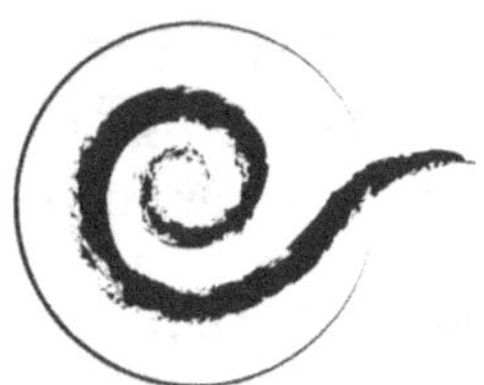

"Krisha - You know you're acting like a VICTIM, right?"

Those words punched me in the gut.

It was the summer of 2019 and I was on a zoom call with a coach friend of mine and she said that to me.

That was probably the worst thing anyone could say about me.

ME? A Victim? No way, I am an empowered goddess!

Also—my mom was the queen of "poor me", and I grew up with that in my face 24/7 so anything that remotely closely resembled the victim mindset had me cringing, angry and defending myself hard.

But it was true.

I was caught in a loop.

I wanted to make a change in my life, it was a big scary one, but nonetheless, a change, and all I kept doing was tell anyone who would listen how awful it was.

"But you don't understand"...was my refrain.

"I just can't"....

"But it's not like that"...

"How?"...

People who would patiently listen to me gripe and complain would tell me how and why, and give me the steps, but my mind would stop listening.

I would immediately go unconscious and not hear a word they said. I would pretend I was listening - "Uh huh, yeah.Ok yes! I will do that!"

But 30 seconds later I'd be like "Hey anyone who will listen, I have this problem and have no clue how to fix it, can someone please save me! You don't understand, I have done ALL the work, I've done EVERYTHING and yet I'm STILL not moving forward. What's it gonna take?"

Which turned into my conversations with God—"How can you be so mean to me? Why are you punishing me? What's wrong with me? I don't get it, what's it gonna take for you to reward my efforts?"

Oh yeah, it was a rich tapestry of Victim Mentality...and I couldn't see it.

So when my coach was like - WAKE THE FUCK UP—I woke up.

Her opinion mattered to me, and I did NOT want to be seen as a victim...so...

I entered the arena of deeper shadow work than I've ever done before.

I was guided by a very powerful mentor who introduced me to Vicky the Victim, my inner little girl who was running my life.

She was everywhere...money, love, sex.

She was this wounded little girl, who had never been taught how to "adult" properly in her life, and instead took the wheel as a child to adult her parent and kept that role into her own adulthood.

There were many areas where I had personal responsibility, wisdom and empowerment, but many more I didn't.

Facing Vicky was not easy, she was hanging on for dear life.

She was my best friend, the person inside of me that gave me an "out", an excuse for not playing bigger, for, well, being a Victim.

We went deep, dark and into some very, very painful and scary moments. Some of them included me punching my own face in a desperate need to be rid of that way of thinking...

It was dark.

And she held on for dear life, because who were "we" without this? Who was I, how was I going to relate, to run my business, to parent without this part of me? What was going to replace her? What if the replacement was WORSE???

Impossible.

What happened instead was a shedding of her, a loosening of her grip as I recognized over and over and over again that I was SAFE, I was LOVED, I was FREE and I was ok to be ME.

I faced the kids that made fun of me in school—like really mean shit.

I faced my mom and we had a great meeting (she was deceased, we had a medium guide us) and I got answers as to why she did what she did to herself.

I looked at how I was showing up as a mother (that was very puke-worthy), and the kinds of men I was allowing between my sheets.

I kept diving deeper and deeper and deeper until there was nothing left.

All that remained was me.

A pure, super shiny, amazing, spark of consciousness.

That's it.

My only job now is to shine this light, be this giant reflection for humanity and remain present enough at all times to soak up the juiciness of this planet.

I retired Vicky sometime in 2020, she now plays and is my creative side, but she no longer comes up and sabotages me the way she used to. She doesn't need to, because I trust myself now, so she doesn't need to "take the wheel" anymore.

She can just breathe, and be there as the purpose she was here to be...enjoy the fuck out of this life, and be an early detection system for me when things are off-kilter (aka red flag detector).

HOW TO SPOT VICTIM MENTALITY

First of all. Nobody likes this topic, it's very confronting to learn you're acting like a victim, especially if you're otherwise a strong, independent and intelligent woman.

I work with women like this every day, and I can spot that victim voice from a million miles away...and almost all of us have it. So there's no judgement here, only a compassionate willingness to grow and learn and love ourselves into aligned harmony and learning to speak our minds without fear or the need to manipulate.

Victim mentality is rife in our society, everywhere you look someone is claiming to be a victim of circumstances, and this is an incredibly disempowering way to live.

I'm not saying there are not legit times where we have been victim to things like assault, racism/discrimination, abuse, natural disasters etc...we need to put that aside.

I'm talking about the victim mindset that we see played out in every single television show and movie, books, and most definitely every reality show out there (it's this narrative that makes those shows so addictive). It shows up in most workplaces, and definitely in families and relationships.

THE DRAMA TRIANGLE

First, we need to learn about the Drama Triangle, a concept developed by Steven Karpman, to demonstrate the Victim, Perpetrator, Saviour loop most of us fall under when we operate out of alignment and in survival mode.

For me, it was all three and each one would come out in different circumstances.

The Victim Voice sounds like this: "But you don't get it. But why? But why not? I don't get it, why me? Why not me? I can't have, I shouldn't, I'm "fine". You want people to read your mind and get upset if they don't. You can't make decisions on your own (you ask for advice from everyone). Can't make decisions for yourself.

The Saviour Voice sounds like this: "Let me do that for you. Sure I have the time (when you don't). Just give it to me, I'll do it. Are you open to some feedback? Can I give you feedback? I'm just trying to help! She doesn't understand, so I'll just do it for her. I'm trying to protect my kids from getting hurt!". This is the classic enabler, and they avoid confrontation.

The Perpetrator Voice sounds like this: "If you really loved me you would. I'm better than her, why does she get him? No, I'm right". Gaslighting (denying the feelings of another). Blame, and fault finding. The classic bully/narcissist.

The first step in any of this work is to become conscious and aware of the words that come out of your mouth and the thoughts in your head. This is where practicing silence when you want to respond (react) comes in, and meditation.

If you hear yourself speaking out these voices (or thinking them), you've done the hardest part: becoming consciously aware of your shadow/subconscious blindspots!!! This is HUGE so don't underestimate it.

The next step is replacing the voice with a new one.

I will say at this point—if there's a part of you that is offended or says "I'm not like this at all"...you're in serious denial.

I am not here to judge or make anyone wrong or feel badly...I am here to shine a light on the shadow so we can turn it into the light. This is a very difficult set of behaviours to admit to, so please have compassion for yourself and be really honest, because the opposite side of the Drama Triangle is where healthy relating and dating really comes in, otherwise you will be caught in a trauma bond with people for the rest of your life and never know how to end it and find truly healthy love.

THE OPPOSITE SIDE OF THE DRAMA TRIANGLE

We have the opportunity to step into something more powerful for ourselves by looking at each side of the triangle and creating its opposite. The opposite side of the Drama Triangle is called **The Empowerment Dynamic** from David Emerald—here's my take on it.

Creator - previously the Victim, the Creator gets to empower themselves to find out how to "save" their own lives and thrive, tap into the power within them already and heal the stories that kept them repressed. Victim is ungrounded feminine energy, and the Creator is the ultimate in Divine Feminine POWER!*

Challenger - previously the Perpetrator, the Challenger gets to set boundaries. The Challenger creates structure (this is healthy masculine energy, by the way), whereas the Perpetrator was all about control (ungrounded masculine energy). I call this **Leader or Warrior or Priestess.** When we are tapped into our own healthy Masculine energy, we are grounded, emotionally safe (no gaslighting!), and have healthy egos (no need to bully) - so we can lead from a place of Divine Masculine POWER!*

Coach - previously the Saviour, the Coach gets to support and guide someone through their own personal empowerment without enabling or taking the power away from the other individual. You resist the urge to run in and solve or save, and instead just listen and only give advice when asked and you give it with zero attachment to whether they take it or not...now THAT is healthy!!!

**A quick note: Divine Masculine & Feminine are spiritual Energies in every human, tree, rock etc on the planet - they are energies, not gender-related. Think of Yin & Yang—it represents the balance of these energies.*

IT'S NEVER TOO LATE TO STEP INTO SOMETHING NEW & POWERFUL!

Within every storm, there is an opportunity to be reborn, and being caught up in the Victim mindset deserves the opportunity to be reborn.

The most difficult part of this work is the personal responsibility piece, especially after a lifetime of seeking outside ourselves for answers.

It was so difficult to face over and over again that I was responsible for my own happiness, it did not feel true to me, it felt like a lie, or that I WAS trying to be responsible but it wasn't happening for me like it was for everyone else. I was deeply convinced that everyone else had this power, but I did not—and this is one of the key identifiers of the Victim voice.

When I was going through healing all of this I also sat with a lot of shame and embarrassment over how I presented myself to my friends and colleagues. There was a period of time where I couldn't face them—I was sure they could see through my facade that I was incapable of making decisions for myself, and I felt incredibly weak, and even meek.

I was out of integrity and felt like an imposter in my work because I was empowering other women to be strong and empowered and there I was still caught in this loop.

It took nearly 2 years of deep shadow work, meditation, journaling and coaching (and loads of breathwork, and tons of time honouring my Divine Feminine and Divine Masculine within) to finally say Bon Voyage to Vicky and her ways.

I kept seeing over and over again how she was running my life into the ground, even though I "knew better". She was choosing men who didn't honour me, where I turned into the victim of their narcissistic (perpetrator) ways. Where I chose "bad boys" who needed "saving", and I would gaslight people who thought differently than I did (mostly because I was never "heard" as a kid, so I yelled louder to get my point across).

That last piece was one of the toughest things I overcame—I had no idea I was doing it consciously. Me??? A Perpetrator??? What???? There is NO WAY I am narcissistic.

Except, I was.

When I saw that shadow behaviour of mine I immediately went into a shame spiral and truly had a Jesus moment with myself.

What I needed to realize was that I COULD have healthy love and communication, and not need to railroad and be right, and to work on my self-worth and self-love first and foremost before stepping one foot back into the dating arena.

I realized my Perpetrator was about winning, and about a toxic need to be desired and recognized because I felt so unloveable and unseen.

So I got to work on loving my own self, honouring myself, winning as myself, seeing my own self first.

I stopped looking outside of myself and every time I had a thought "Oh I should ask so and so how to help me with this" (victim needing to be saved), I would immediately stop, take a breath, and ask: how can I help myself?

I stopped trying to help other people without them asking me first, and even then I hold back unless they are a client who has hired me to coach them.

And I most definitely stopped trying to be right and not railroad others who had a different opinion than me.

And over time, with lots of patience, compassion and also mixed with the deep dark I told you in the beginning, I finally emerged on the other side, free of Vicky's grasp, free of her incessant need to run the show and empowered as my higher self, here to guide and lead, here to embody the Divine Feminine and Masculine and to honour my body, mind and soul.

So many of us have had traumas in our lives, really unfortunate things happen to us by adults or abusers that we truly were victim to. This trauma creates a body language that keeps us stuck in old loops and patterns of survival to keep us safe - especially if that abuse started in childhood - and it can take a lot of work to remove yourself from the grasp of this state.

I am a survivor of trauma and have helped many people heal through it by using the gifts I have, and I know that with a combined approach of body, mind and soul techniques, each of us can have the chance to shed the survival based patterns and truly become the Creator of our own lives.

Body - learning somatic and embodiment techniques to teach your body that it's safe in the here and now, use your senses and nourish it with the right foods, movement and environment (and people!). Tantra practices are great for the body!

Mind - work on the neural pathways and cognitive mindset loops with a therapist, hypnotist or other certified mindset guide to train your brain into new thought patterns to tone down the panic-based thoughts that put you into survival mode, and thus having you act like a victim, perp or saviour.

Soul - learning who you ARE before all the conditioning by using something like Human Design and spending time alone with yourself and getting to know the YOU that's in there somewhere. Energy work is great for this, shaman, soul retrieval, akashic records.

These three elements are part of my daily practices and how I support my clients as well, otherwise if one is missing, your healing never truly feels complete. Something always feels missing. You feel like you're seeking.

And this seeking is what keeps us stuck in that Drama Triangle ~ so if you're finding yourself aware but not sure what to do, ask yourself these three questions and then go out there and get the support you need!

1. Am I always in my head? Do I eat healthy foods and move my body daily? How overwhelmed and stressed do I feel on average?
2. How loud is that judgy voice in my head? Why do I keep sabotaging myself? How hard am I on myself and others? What are the stories running in my head? Am I creating drama that isn't there?
3. Do I know my purpose/why I'm here? Do I trust the voice inside me (can I even hear it)? Am I living the life I really want or am I playing a role for everyone else?

Wherever you are on your journey, know that you're in exactly the right place. I'm 45 and figured this stuff out after two failed marriages...it's never too late! My life now is so rich in possibility, my relationships are balanced and loving. My purpose is clearly laid out and I am LIVING life to the fullest, every single day. I can honestly say that I am in love with myself and that inner judge is a thing of the past.

As I shared, I overcame a lot to get here - and all it took was a willingness to face what needed to be faced, learn to love the discomfort, stop numbing out, and open myself up to receive all the amazing things this world has for all of us.

If I can do this...so can you!

Isn't it time you quiet the storm in you? It's time to be re-born, to Re-Member who you are and live out your purpose!

KRISHA YOUNG

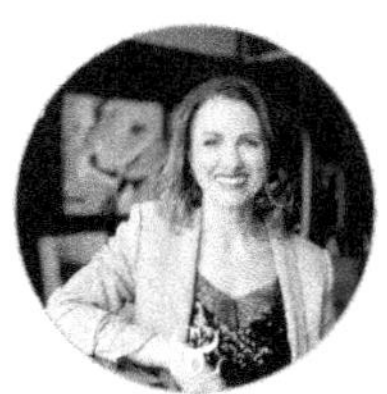

Mind UnFucker & Worthiness Coach. Krisha teaches women how to have healthy relationships, starting with themselves. Her specialty is Pattern Release Coaching for high-performing women healing from self-betrayal.

Krisha knows what happens when we betray ourselves and has devoted her life to help women heal their heart, feel peace and calm and feel sexier inside and out.

In addition to being an entrepreneur, coach, serial podcaster, published author and mom of two boys, Krisha speaks a unique language of transformation developed through years of deep study and synthesizing modalities including Human Design, Holistic Nutrition, Somatic Practices, Tantra and Kundalini.

Krisha does not play small, and she will share with you what YOUR unique gifts are and how you can best use and develop them to have the relationship and life of your dreams.

You can find Krisha and her work here:

Website: krishayoung.com

Krisha's Podcasts

Instagram: @thekrishayoung

9

A SPIRITUAL GIRL IN A DYSFUNCTIONAL WORLD

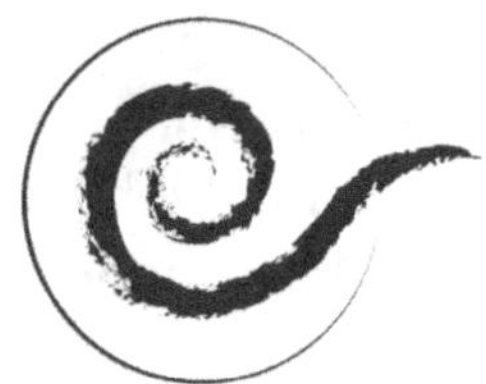

Every person has a story to tell. No matter how big or small. I am writing this story for myself but also for you. Before I share something I always think about what I want to mediate. Will it be helpful or inspiring to others? Could it ignite the flame of hope or recognition in another person? If I can transmit the feeling to just one person, that there is always a reason to carry on, then I have succeeded. Sometimes we have to show ourselves vulnerable for the sake of empowering others and awake empathy among each other.

It was the blizzard of 1979. It was one of the greatest storms of the century. Southern Sweden was more or less a catastrophic area. For some reason the little starseed thought it was the perfect moment to start her life on planet Earth. Patience was never one of her strong sides. It was a miracle that her mother managed to get to the hospital since the snow was covering houses and cars and the wind was too bad for sending out a helicopter. It was the first time that she cheated death and opened her turquoise eyes for the very first time.

The second time she cheated death was in the spring of 1979. She came from a family of farmers and during the fertile time of the year they had to work around the clock to survive on the income that the land could bring. So there was no chance for her mother to be a stay at home mom, even when the little girl was lying in the cradle. So one frisky spring day in April, she had to bring her in the wagon out on the fields. While her parents and grandparents were cultivating the fields, the strong winds were rocking her to sleep. For anyone who has been in Sweden, you know that they can be biting cold at this time of year. A while afterwards the child seemed to lack energy to do almost anything. Luckily she had an uncle who was a physician and his immediate reaction was that the girl had to go to a hospital right away. Before she even reached the hospital elevator, she became unconscious. The team of doctors and nurses desperately tried to cure her but the medications were ineffective. Her little body was covered with tubes and the needles made the fragile vessels in her head burst. She had double-sided pneumonia with a twenty-five percent chance of surviving. Her family was prepared for the unavoidable and the priest was called upon. Then somehow she miraculously healed. She was in and out of hospital for the next year and celebrated her first birthday there. The hospital was her second home for some time due to her brittle health. Her near crossing over probably helped her develop a high sensibility to things around her. This event became a reminder that she got another shot at life and that she always had to carry on no matter what.

She grew up realizing that she was not an ordinary child, with the pros and cons of that fact. Growing up on a farm made her form a special relationship with animals from a very early age. She gained their trust and they gained hers. She noticed that extraordinary things could happen in the presence of love. She used to bring home injured animals. She bathed them, dried them and gave them all of her love and caring. She also noticed that when they were hurting, she could stroke them or hold her hand over them and they seemed to recover after that. She had no idea how it happened. As a child you don't think much about how things happen. It just became something natural for her. Of course it didn't always work out. That is how nature works. Life has its reasons.

Like her grandmother she got premonitions about things that were about to happen, everything from natural disasters, people crossing over, everyday events or just like a sense of knowingness of people or what they were about to say. Her grandmother was an extraordinary woman, an iron lady who wasn't afraid of anything or anyone but she spoke little of everything that she had experienced. It must have been hard for her growing up when society was different.

Since the little girl had no siblings and since her parents were working a lot, she spent a lot of time on her own and she was more or less brought up by her grandparents. Their early and sudden crossing over was probably one of the greatest sorrows of her life. The family she ended up in was dysfunctional. She had a harsh upbringing which didn't leave any room for tears or for being weak. Making mistakes could lead to problems sitting down in her school chair because of the pain and her red ears were burning like fire. She can still remember one of her birthday parties where she got humiliated in front of her friends when she got spanked, flew across the room and tripped into a radiator.

She never felt she could ever please her father, no matter what she did, and she spent half of her lifetime proving herself worthy to him, consciously or unconsciously. Already from an early age his little empathetic girl got her heart broken into a million pieces. She felt she was never enough and spent many nights crying herself to sleep. Her sensitive mother tried her best to take care of the girl while living in a dysfunctional marriage. The daughter became the greatest joy and love of her life, although most of the time it was the little girl who had to take care of her mother. The little starseed had a rough start adjusting here although she handpicked her parents herself. They tried their best, she supposes, from their personal skills and level of consciousness. But naturally it affected her sense of self-worth and she never got a sound concept of what a relationship should be like. Despite this, she loves them very dearly and of course there are still endless things about them that she is grateful for. The other side of the coin is that she learned to depend only on herself, skills that would serve her well in the future. Three apples high, she managed herself, school and learned to make her own money doing heavy work on the farm during the summer holidays.

What she hid from the world for most of her life was the fact that she was struggling with anxiety, which many times goes hand in hand with being an empath, with high sensibility, in combination with feeling unsafe as a child. It was something she was not proud of. Instead she had always played a role of being strong because that was something that was rewarded when being a youngster. The anxiety also escalated into severe depressions and already at a young age she spent a lot of time thinking about death. She was plagued by seeing all the suffering in this world, including her own, and she remembered asking God to relocate her somewhere else where she belonged because she couldn't bear to live in it any longer. The thing about anxiety or depression is that you suffer so badly that you want to crawl out of your own skin, sometimes without even knowing why. That constant worry that is nagging inside of you and the feeling that you want to flee all the time and wanting to be anywhere but in the situation you are in at that moment. To cope with herself, she fled into self- destructive behaviours. Early on she refused to eat and as a young woman it continued with heavy partying. Increased drinking became the cure for the emptiness in her heart. Finally it became more and more frequent and she realized she had to make a final break with alcohol. Later on she came to understand that her emotions were sort of on the outside of her body. When she was growing up, no one had come across the word HSP (Highly Sensitive Person). As time went by she learned that the various feelings she had weren't necessarily her own and she had suffered a whole lifetime before realizing this. She had been sad without even really knowing why. Even though she was a happy child with many friends she was unwell and couldn't hold her guard up which led to bullying, more depression and attendance problems.. So the little empath got her heart broken over and over again because it resonated with the feelings of being unwanted and wrong that was imprinted in her already being a toddler.

She always had great love for this world and its inhabitants. When someone else suffered, she suffered as well and most of her life she avoided conflicts for the sake of peace. Due to her healing abilities she often attracted people with great need of healing into her life. This is probably why she came across people with great darkness inside of them because they are often drawn to empaths who can help them replace their emptiness with light. She was always filled with the feeling that her love could heal everything and everyone no matter what the cost. She was having a Messiah Complex and delusions of grandeur. This is the great lesson for empaths. They get consumed by the cause and forget that if they go down with the fall there is nothing more to save. Not even themselves. This is not self-love. If we let other people drag us down we won't be able to save or be of use to anyone else.

The result was that in her youth, destruction also came in the form of relationships, dominated by endless conflicts and betrayals. Maybe because she had never learned what a healthy relationship should be like. Sometimes she felt like almost living in a prison, where she constantly had to find coping mechanisms and strategies to avoid or settle conflicts. She weighed her words and actions on a scale. Eventually she went silent. The odd thing is that she didn't realize herself when she had given away her voice and life space. She thought she could handle it, that she knew what she was doing. That nothing could get to her. But of course it did. Piece by piece she lost her self-esteem. It took divine intervention to help her understand that it was finally time to leave and move forward. Her health was at the absolute bottom but there were still storms to come. Once she thought she had found a safe haven, it was really just another delusion. The white knights that promised to treat her well after her past experiences were always new dead ends. It was a constant downgoing spiral with conflicts, infidelities and lies.

So early in life she let people take advantage of her good heart. One of the greatest betrayals she was put through in life, from her experience, was when people criticized her persona or her beliefs. She was mocked for her spirituality and she shed a lot of tears, especially when being criticized by people she loved. But she didn't let that criticism change her beliefs one bit and one day it couldn't get to her anymore. It is not always pain on the outside that hurts the most, it is when the thought that you might not be worthy of love starts to grow inside of you.

So the starseed had her own personal experience of the painful part of life in the third dimension. Broken from the inside, she tried not to show it to the outside world, always trying to put on a smile as a barrier. But because she stayed focused on her starseed mission of unconditional love and peace she could also experience the sweetness of life. The joys and love of this dimension. It would not have been possible without the duality of this world. She also realized that you can only be your own saviour and that we get presented to the same situations until the lesson is learned.

If you can relate in any way to this story you have to take precautions to protect your precious heart. Having that said, for the same reason that you might be used for your loving heart, you can also use your heart as your superpower. If you can realize what a great gift you have in your hands you will know your heart is your greatest asset in this world. Part of taking back my power has been through forgiveness. Today I hold no grudges and I only use my stories to demonstrate how you can grow from your experiences. If you are stuck in anger and resentment you will never have full access to your energy and your mind will always dwell in the past and prevent you from living in the present. People cross our paths for a reason and I don't believe in evil persons, only various types of consciousness. The final stage of healing your past is when you can see God in every person you meet, even in the people that have hurt you. That is why I can love everyone, regardless of what they might have done, although it is not a physical love but a universal one.

When I took back my power I gained access to my true potential. All I own in this world and all that I have accomplished is because of me and it makes me feel truly powerful and independent. I try not to linger anymore in the pain that I have experienced. I have reached a point in my life where I realize that all experiences serve a perfect purpose, even if it is not always easy to see or understand. It is up to us how we choose to manage those experiences. It is our responsibility how we treat people, even the ones that have hurt us. I don't share my stories to play a victim or to point fingers at anyone. I share my stories because I want to be understood, transparent, to make people feel that there is always hope and you are never alone. I don’t believe that there is a single thing in this life that you can't get through or at least to learn to live with. I believe that we write our own manuscripts, filled with karmic events to make us grow wiser. I am now pursuing my dreams and my heart's deepest desires on a whole other level than before and I no longer compromise with myself. I see all people I meet and all the events that present themselves before me as masterclasses in the evolvement of my soul. Every hardship that I experience, somehow makes the compassion and love in my heart grow even stronger.

I strongly believe that things happen to us for a reason. Maybe you experienced something because later on, that experience was supposed to help someone else. So I have learned to turn things around. I work daily with my weaknesses to improve myself. Before I didn't like myself and tried to suppress the real me. My big lesson in life has been to start loving myself and to realize that the combination of being a spiritual sensitive empath, really makes me an asset in building a new world. When I started out on my spiritual path for real, between ten and twenty years ago I realized why it had been so hard for me to adjust to life on this planet. I learned to know my true self, my origin and my real mission on earth, to help people heal and align with the frequency of love. It was also the cure I needed for my own healing. I have replaced self-destruction with self-love. I am also here to study new things and transform that knowledge into tools for helping myself and others. The greatest wisdom I gained from the experiences that took me from the darkest places to the unconditional love in my heart. When you think you know everything, I think that calls for a reality check. After years of meditation and expanding my mind I have been able to learn to cope with my anxiety and my past. We are who we are for a reason and we should be proud of ourselves, with all of our flaws and imperfections. We all have our challenges in life, otherwise we would not stay humble and empathetic.

Today I work holistically with giving services in healing and herbal medicine therapy. I also teach mindfulness, mediation, Qi Gong and coach others for personal development and spiritual growth. I also work with empowering women through teaching mindset, self-defence, coaching for better self-esteem, to feel safe and confident in society. My mission in life is to bring as much love into this world as possible and help people transform their lives through fulfilling their life's purpose and achieve better health within body, mind, soul and spirit. I am at full disposal to help you, based on the knowledge and the consciousness that I possess today. I want to help you see the divine in yourself that I can see in you.

Every person has a story. I am a full-fledged survivor and a warrior of love. I am stormborn and I have been mastering storms ever since. There will always be new storms and hardships during our lifetime but once you see that they serve as a purpose for your growth, you can learn to bend and dance with them. Are you ready to take my hand, stand in your power and swirl with them now?

LENA SVENSSON

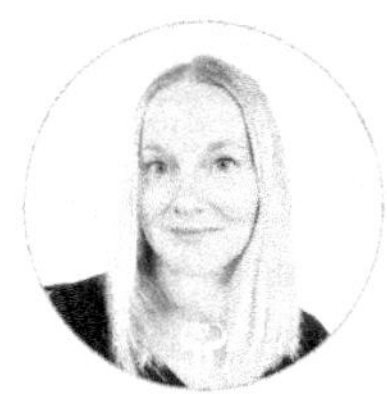

Lena, aka Chiqui, is an old soul who has as her greatest mission in life to bring as much love into this world as possible. She is passionate about helping you become the best version of yourself, grow from your experiences and make you shine like the star you really are.

Lena is a trained healer but has been a natural healer since she was a child. She is a herbal medicine therapist and works as a holistic health advisor, since she believes in treating body, mind, soul and spirit as a whole to gain optimal health. Lena also works and holds diplomas in areas such as mindfulness, meditation, stress coping, qi gong, life coaching and spiritual coaching. In addition to this, she also works with empowering women, which includes instruction in self-defence and teaching strategies for women to feel powerful and safe in society.

Contact information:
https://linktr.ee/LenaChiquiSvensson

10

RECOVERY IS ALWAYS POSSIBLE

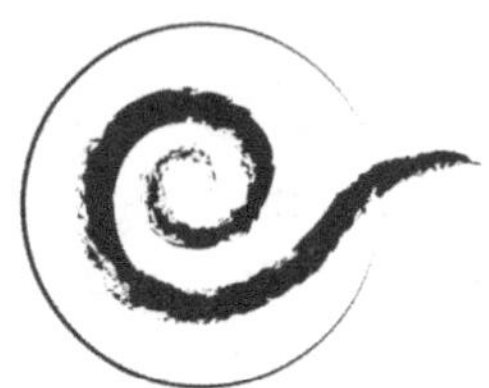

"Freak. Weirdo. Outsider. Misfit. Black sheep. Worthless. No good piece of shit. No one wants to be with me, not really, and I know it. No one will ever love me, not if they truly knew who I really am. So be a smart girl, and cover up. Take everything down a notch, don't be too much or too little, don't laugh so hard, and for Gods sake, be feminine, like a REAL woman! And don't be yourself".

Those were all mine. My inner voices. I've heard them for as long as I can remember, always. Sometimes from other people, mostly when I grew up, which is really common when you're a child, but I was the one who kept talking to myself in such a mean and destructive way, putting myself down, and I didn't even reflect, I wasn't aware. I didn't believe in myself in the slightest. Not even one little bit. That was my secret. No one could know. I was so ashamed of myself, and ashamed of my appearance, my body, my goofy way, everything. It's impossible to live with those voices in your head, never keeping quiet, always feeding you with lies, day and night. Eventually it becomes your truth, and that is so excruciatingly painful, that you will do anything to make it go away. And I did. I certainly did.

I tried to make it go away in every way I could think of. Alcohol, prescription drugs, food, sugar, sex, attention seeking behaviour, you name it. When I was only fourteen years old, I realised something that was going to be very important to me for the next sixteen years. The constant war in my head, my tormenting inner voices, my pain and my anxiety actually could be silenced! I found a new best friend, called alcohol. From the first time that I drank it, I became its prisoner. How I loved that I could finally be happy! Feel calm, have good vibes, and be that funny girl that everyone loved, the girl I never had the guts to be, when I was sober. I found my solution, and that's where it all began, at my cousins wedding, almost thirty years ago. I was a tall, blond, shy girl in a red dress, only fourteen years old, and I was so proud to be mistaken for an adult, drinking red wine for the first time ever.

The rush I felt from the alcohol was magic. Pure magic running through my veins, making me strong, brave and in peace. The rush went away quickly, they always do. But I wanted to feel that again, at every cost. And why wouldn't I? I had never felt so free! I wanted that freedom back.

Alcohol is a true magician. It makes stuff disappear, for real! It makes anxiety go away, fear, hunger, shyness, shame, everything I wanted to get rid of. But, in the long run, it also makes your self-worth go away. It makes your life more and more empty, preventing you from having intimate relationships. It takes your money away, your dignity and your ability to have a meaningful life. It takes everything, until what remains of you is emptiness. A frozen soul, with no dreams or hope left. It takes some time, of course, to get to the point where you are completely drained, broken and depressed. For me, I managed to get through my teens and my early twenties before I was really hooked. At twenty-five, that's were it got to the point of no return. A downward spiral, that could only end in chaos and despair.

I easily fell in love lots of times, at least, that was what I thought. I got into many destructive and harmful relationships, lots of one night stands, still searching for love, something good. I loved that intense feeling when I felt attracted to someone, and I truly believed that what I felt was love, falling in love. I did confuse intensity with intimacy, I had no idea there even was a difference at that time. I had to learn the hard way and the long way what it is really like to have an intimate relationship. I wasn't ready to find out until I had over ten years of unbroken recovery. I was confused, uneducated of living and too scared.

That's why I ended up with a man who was a sex and porn addict. I tried so hard to fit in with someone, to get some love, some attention, so I made myself the one he wanted. I did everything he asked for, day and night, no matter how little I slept or how bad it made me feel. He didn't ever hurt me physically, but I did let him do stuff to me, in grave pain, but I never said anything. I did subconsciously decide to just bare with it. Convinced myself I wanted the same, that I liked it too. I became as much of a sex addict myself, forcing my body into climaxing all the time, even if it felt completely wrong and I was hurting myself deeply, but it no longer mattered to me. It took me a couple of years to get out of this relationship, but when I did, I couldn't bare to touch my body. Not ever, if I could avoid it. Not even in the shower, to wash myself. I felt so nauseous when I touched myself and my vagina, that I just couldn't do it. For several weeks the only way to wash was to just rinse myself with water. I have shared this with only two or three people in this world so far, but it needs to get out there. This is not my shame to bear.

I continued to drink heavily during my last years with active addiction. I always had some excuse, if I had company, hey—it's party time! It's time to celebrate life! It's frickin' Tuesday! I never took any pills when I was together with friends, that was just for me, I was still content with free access to alcohol. It still gave me some peace, even if I felt like shit the day after. There were always more to drink!

One day, out for lunch with a friend, this cute guy came to our table, talking to her. I instantly wanted him. I had to have him! Today I can obviously see how sick I was, but that was the only way I knew at the time. When he left, she told me that he was a member of Narcotics Anonymous. Great, I thought! Now I know where to find him! I found out where the meeting was, and I went. I have no idea how I had the guts to just go down in that basement that dark night in February 2008, but I did. He wasn't there. But, I stayed through the whole meeting.

The only thing I remember is that all the people welcomed me with such warmth, and that they read to me, a text called "the newcomer", from a little white book. I heard but one thing, "no one enters the doors to NA without a reason". It scared me to death. I was there to find a cute guy, nothing else! But I stayed. And I kept coming back. My friends from this group told me, years after, that I actually spoke for several minutes, laughing, crying, and I don't remember a single moment, not even to this day. I started going to those meetings regularly. Didn't drink or take pills. At first I behaved much like an animal, I didn't want anyone to see any of my human weaknesses. I felt so very uncomfortable with anyone seeing me eating, sleeping or crying, that I had to use the bathroom. Even yawning I didn't do in public at first. But, I went to meetings, listened to others, talking and sharing about their lives, their feelings,

and I shared mine. I started to enjoy it, and best of all, I didn't feel alone anymore. In that room, with those people, I finally felt normal, for the first time in my life.

Two days from my first recovery badge, 30 days of sobriety, I decided that I was well, I wasn't sick and I wasn't an addict. How could I be, being sober for 28 days? I decided to celebrate. That celebration did not end until two weeks later. Two whole weeks of constant drinking. Can a normal, healthy person really do that? Of course not.

That's where I was when I had to make my biggest choice so far. Did I want to live—or die? I gave it a good thought, and realised I didn't really want to die, but I didn't want to live in the way I did either, so what was left to do? I decided to cut myself. I was delirious, so I couldn't think straight. I decided to cut myself, bad enough, but not lethal, so that maybe someone could save me.

My legs. Big arteries, so there will be lots of blood, but maybe it won't kill me. I can cut myself, and immediately call for help. That was my plan. So, I reached for my biggest kitchen knife. I used a grinding steel and started to make it real sharp. It felt like trance, watching that knife, listening to the scratching sound it made when I sharpened the blade. All of a sudden, I heard a sound. Next thing I know, one of my cats sat next to me, making sounds in her cat way. That woke me up, and I dropped the knife on the floor. I cried for hours that day.

Two days later, I was going to a meeting with my mom and some of our friends, a military group for women. The meeting was not far from where I lived, so I decided to take the bike. Getting on the bike, I realised that my hands were shaking, and I couldn't get them to stop. What was happening to me? I stared at my hands. And then, I realised. I finally realised, that the reason my hands were shaking, was that I was an addict, an alcoholic who needed her drink. It felt like my world fell apart, and my body cracked from the inside, like this insight had broken me.

Somehow I got through the meeting, but afterwards I went straight to the pub. I ordered whiskey and beer, and sat down to drink. I drank a lot that night, and I started smoking again, nothing mattered anymore. I just had to gather all the courage available to me, as I knew I had to ask for help.

I have always been quite a private person, so I managed to hide my addiction from everyone in my life. I still don't understand how, but I did. Of course, some people told me I drank too much sometimes, but that was it. I convinced everyone that I was A-OK. And, I'm sure that's how it looked. I had an apartment, a car, I studied full time, had friends, no trouble with money or the police I had what you can call "a normal life". But, whenever I was alone, and I was alone a lot, I drank. Not just like that, but in a way I felt I could control. I had one rule I never intended to break. No drinking before 6 pm. Not once.

And no drinking and driving. I followed that rule for a long time, but as my addiction escalated, I started to break more and more rules, laws, moral codes, everything. You see, eventually you get emotionally numb. Alcohol and other drugs do that to you, that's why I used them anyway. The more you hurt people around you and hurt yourself, the more you have to numb yourself in the long run. No one can cope with that amount of pain, if you don't numb yourself with something. I broke all of my rules as my addiction got worse. All of them. I was drinking around the clock. I broke laws, I was driving drunk. I was constantly lying. Manipulating people to get what I wanted. I was full of shame, guilt, anxiety, fear and grief. But I couldn't stop myself. Everything just kept getting worse, and there was nothing I could do about it. I was a slave to alcohol, and totally under its spell.

The only thing I wanted was to get high, drunk, and pass out. Not feel anything, to get away. I often passed out on the floor and woke up hours later. I had lots of really big bruises, caused by falls, and accidents. One time some girls in my class saw my back. They were horrified... Half of my back was actually black, from a huge bruise that I got when I fell down from a dresser, on a stool. I didn't remember anything, but I figured it out.

It all went so far, that in the end, nothing was left of the real me. I was trying to hide behind my fake smile, my way of making others feel good, but still hoping that someone, someday, would see me. See the real me, and actually want to get to know me. See some worth in me, that I didn't see. And come to my rescue. That, of course, never happened. I didn't know then, but with time I got to understand that the only rescuer ever, was going to be me. Just me, and only me.

I called a good friend of mine. Told him the truth, that I was slowly killing myself drinking, that I couldn't stop on my own. Thirty minutes later, he was there. Got me home, and the next day he helped me get to the nearest hospital. I was so scared when I rang the bell at the right section, the locked floor, Detoxification. Mostly I was scared that they wouldn't let me in. "Nope, no place for you here, go home!" But, they didn't. Of course they didn't. I signed in for a voluntary detox. In there for six days another journey began. The real journey.

To get clean and stay clean, you have to understand addiction, what it is, and the enormous power addiction has on human beings. It's not difficult to get clean. On the contrary, what is difficult, is to stay clean. You need to learn that, really learn, both emotionally and theoretically, and it's very hard. It takes a lot of time to really get to know yourself again, and understand the why. The why is so very important! The key to recovery.

What is addiction? Drugs? The need to use it? No. The drugs, the behaviour, that's only symptoms which hide the real cause. Drugs are used to FEEL differently, to change an emotion to something else, or remove it. Addiction is being uncapable to feel, handle and take care of your own feelings. If you don't suffer, you don't need to numb yourself, right? That's why addiction is an emotional and spiritual disease. All of this is my own personal beliefs, and I'm only speaking for myself and what I have learned along the way.

My real journey didn't start until I rid myself of all sorts of drugs and behaviours that was bad for me, and that took me years. First, I had to learn to live without drugs and alcohol, that was the easy part, really. But then, I had to learn to live again. On life's own terms, that is. Get to know myself, who I really was. Invite other people into my life, have intimate and true relationships, all my biggest wishes and fears. Luckily, I had great help along the way!

This is not a journey you can or should do on your own, that's not the way. If you don't step out of your comfort zone, you can't have the changes that you long for in your life.

Today I am thankful for my fantastic rescue. Was I rescued by a knight on a white horse? Nope. By God, a higher power, love, or whatever you would like to call it? Partially, yes, because I believe that my journey through hell was meant to be, and to make me, both who I am today, and who I will be tomorrow. I do believe in something good, something powerful.

However, most of it was my own creation. Many years of really hard work, process after process, and the thing with me is—I never stop. I want to be better, more, know more, understand more, peel off more layers and get even closer to my core. When I'm writing this, I have been in recovery for a little more than thirteen years, and if I continue working on myself, I can stay sober. I'm still on my journey, and I will be until the day I die. Today my passion is about giving what I once was given, to others. I have the deepest understanding that what I've been through, I can use in favour for others, particularly my sisters in this world. I see a lot of people who need us surviving warriors, who need us to be their guides and show them the way out of the darkness. That is my true calling, my passion, my internal drive. I am the Swedish amazon warrior, the protector of other women. I always will be. Remember, sisters and brothers, darkness is a natural part of life. Darkness is a gateway to the light, so don't fear it! Embrace it, get to know your own darkness, and you will have a good life. I don't know anything about a happy ending. But, at least I finally got my happy beginning.

LIZA BUSTAD

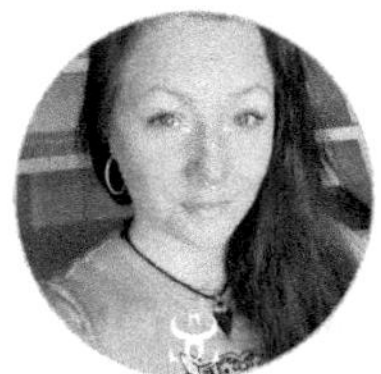

Liza is an artist of life, an educated healer and a survivor of serious addiction. She has over twelve years of experience sponsoring other women in recovery.

Liza has her roots deep down in the earth, seeking wisdom in nature and in life's own ways. Her lifepath has been anything but straight, still she is very grateful for everything she has experienced. She wouldn't be the person she is today, if it wasn't for all the hard life lessons she had to learn. By learning and experiencing for herself, she can also pass her knowledge on to other women with addiction and codependency.

Liza has a diploma in spiritual healing, and is currently educating in MI – Motivational Interviewing, to reach even more people in need of guidance. Her true passion is to help people find their way back to life.

E-mail: liza_bustad@yahoo.se

Instagram: www.instagram.com/comfortzonewithliza

11

BORN WITH A CURSE

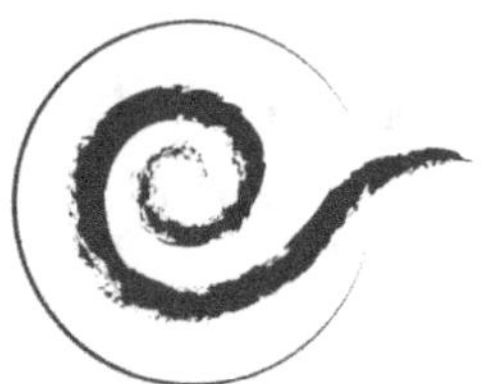

My start in life was dramatic. No one in my family knew the curse that had been placed on me from the start and that would affect the inner structure of the family. I was incarnated with hooks attached to my crown chakra with the initiation that I was deprived. There was no chance to escape the plans of the demonic energies for my life. Their plan was diabolical and cruel. I was completely unaware of my power and strength and what it aroused in those who were not born with the gift. Demonic energies choose their victims and I was one of them, forever doomed to be their favourite and prey. They loved to humiliate me.

I tried to take in what she was telling me. The words flowed towards me like a spring flood.

Powerful and determined in its direction to reach me. I tried to gather my thoughts. It sounded completely incomprehensible. At the same time, everything fell into place. All that could not be touched in my life. That which was not comprehensible. How it became more and more obvious that something outside of me affected me. These negative poison arrows I tried to shield myself from that were aimed at me. How the vicious slander against me from a certain person affected me more negatively than I was aware of. My aggressive desperation. How my life just spun around in an ever wilder and more destructive dance every year. A dance I had become aware of. A ring dance that was not mine, but whose was it? What was it that controlled me? My fragile self-confidence and even weaker core. Years in therapy to find an explanation. Attachment problems The horse accident in my youth that caused deep wounds I have not processed. A fragile self. A weak self. A self that I have tried to strengthen through inner and outer training. How my inability to stick together at times was palpable. At the same time, there was a voice inside me, weak and barely audible: "You are not hopeless". A voice that became more and more persistent, more powerful and in the end, I had to listen to that voice deep inside of me, from the depths of my inner being. There was something wrong with my life.

Reality always surprises me. It turned out that reality was something completely different from what I ever could have imagined in my wildest imagination. I became ice cold when the realization fell into place and at the same time as I was filled with a force I decided that enough is enough. The game has been going on long enough, far too long due to my inability to set boundaries, that I have been permissive and tolerant of her at times excessive behaviour. Had I known about the existence of the phenomenon, I would have put a stop to it many years ago. If my parents had known, they would have closed the door to this person already in their youth when she penetrated our home and my energies and then manipulated my whole family and especially me with deep-laid evil. I was the target, the rest was just a backdrop to get me where she wanted.

My whole life was so fraught with misunderstandings and loneliness. An emotional mess that I tried to get through as best as I could. Year after year. Situations were repeated. Lessons learned. A new round. How I repeatedly fell with the thought; I can not take it. Not again.

Over and over again. But I always got to the surface again, even though my longing was always distorted to being rejected again.

Where my longing for love only ended in superficial friendships and love relationships that were doomed from the beginning. Something was wrong. How at times I found myself in bottomless despair where my thoughts and emotional life was a single chaos. Like a leaf in the wind, like a plastic duck on the open sea. A constant groping for something to hold on to.

The best thing is to just turn my back on everything. Stop croaking, stop pretending, stop explaining, stop trying to get my friends to understand. To take off my blindfold and look myself deep in the eyes. To meet my wounds openly and honestly. These people I have surrounded myself with year after year, the ones I called my friends. A heavy insight. Is this it? My inner emptiness that led me astray all my adult life. Then something started to shine inside of me. I thanked my lucky star for getting an eye-opener now, not in the future or maybe never. There are those who die of negativity. Those who never come to insight. My inner self was filled with gratitude for not having these people in my life anymore.

> "I had disappeared for good, and the ease with which it happened
>
> had made it clear to me how shallow my relationships
>
> with all these people had been."
>
> -Siri Hustvedt.

All mixed messages over the years. The bullshit about me that never reached my ears, but were like invisible poison arrows towards me. Never anything concrete until now. The energy bonds were clear to those who have the ability. The woman in the United States wondered what I had done to upset this person so much. I said: nothing! she answered; this woman is completely obsessed with controlling your energies.

She was amazed at the creature I had after me and with the frenzy she repeatedly sent curses at me. Her skill as a magician was due to her accuracy. Strong intention if you will. My feelings were the catalyst. She hated me for a reason I do not understand and do not intend to waste any energy trying to understand. The woman in the United States took an apple as a comparison so that I would understand that this person's interior was so beyond help that she compared it to a rotten apple. She was as incomprehensible as I was to this person's inner decay and evil. I was incomprehensible to how different healers I have had contact with over the years could have missed these destructive energies I was exposed to.

" How have they been able to miss all this!"

I exclaimed in horror. The steep downhill of recent years, both physically and mentally, had led me to alternative forms of therapy as modern healthcare only wanted to prescribe medication.

" Ordinary mediums do not have an understanding of the deep threads of Witchcraft. Spider magic is an ancient variant of Witchcraft that is almost forgotten in our modern society".

Through my own research, I came to the conclusion that shamans still have knowledge of these different variants of entities that can affect those who do not have control over their energy field. Violations of power, similar to infectious diseases, often occur in urban areas where the population is dense. According to shamanism, this is because people, without knowing it, possess the possibility of harming others with outbursts of their personal power when they come to a state of lack of emotional balance, such as anger. When we talk about someone who radiates hostility, it is a latent expression of the shamanic view. A shaman would say that it is dangerous not to know anything about shamanic principles. When you are as ignorant as I was, you do not know how to protect yourself from the intrusion of hostile energy, let alone that the phenomenon exists. People are generally unaware that someone can actually consciously send destructive energies towards someone, so-called curses, and cause great harm to the person in question.

I see myself as the involuntary nurse. My journey as a professional nurse has been shaky since the beginning and I have questioned much of what has happened within the walls of modern healthcare over the years. I have devoted an entire professional life to a job I am extremely ambivalent about. It took many years before I could put my finger on what it was that did not suit either me or the profession I chose. The work environment in closed ward is so skewed that it is difficult to find the right words and the right forum for what is wrong.

Today it is even more infected and the focus has shifted to whether you are for or against vaccines. A polarization that one did not think was possible has arisen in our society where the issue is about our human rights and our freedom of choice. If you are unaware of that you are an empath, your innate gifts can create more misfortune than happiness.

I missed words for a long time to describe my experience. If you suffer from cancer, it is an obvious diagnosis, but when I tell those around me that I was exposed to black magic and have been for many years, they backfire! For a while, my need to tell was endless as I was in some kind of state of shock. That it was a person near me who did it. A person like you and me. At the family party. In the circle of friends. Married sisters-in-law or brothers-in-law. People who lived by a double agenda. With fake smiles and hidden agenda, they took the opportunity to have fun activating the negative energy substance that housed my body so it hijacked my personality so that I got blacked out and did not remember anything except that they took turns blocking my energies. When I tried to convey the reality I had gained insight into, to those around me, it became difficult for them. Their rallies were palpable.

"Are you sure you have received the right help?"

"What is that shaman trying to make you believe? She's fooling you for money, beware!"

"Are you now trying to use this as an excuse for your life not turning out as you intended?"

I felt misunderstood by my closest friends. That was before I realized I was surrounded by black magicians. All my friends were around me for one reason only. I was surrounded by bloodthirsty wolves. It is not possible to explain to someone who has not been in those energies and to try to get understanding from those who were involved in the act. It was bound to fail as they saw it as their life task to block my flow of life and my life force. The grip that the negative energies have on you is only understood by oneself when they begin to be cleared away. I was unknowingly drawn to these energy vampires long after I was clean. The purifications were a steel bath and sometimes I doubted my own sanity but the shaman's words echoed in my head:

"You are not mentally ill. It all depends on this! The images and emotions must come to the surface in order to disappear. The only way to get rid of it, is to face what you have been exposed to."

I pulled myself together and made a decision. The film strip that was rolled up in my mind made me see the connections clearly. The world is not what they want us to believe. What do we really know about the world we live in? To be met by the sceptical looks and defensive speeches of those around us hurt and their words rang in my ears:

"There is no human being who can be so cruel, right?"

I felt infinitely alone in my situation. Exposed and questioned. I was looking for methods and contexts to deal with the world I had woken up to. All the energy attacks and blockages of my life flow had damaged my health in various ways.

The doctor at the healthcare barely looked at me. He didn't even check the basic things that could be possible to follow up as my vital parameters; blood pressure, heart rate, temperature and weight. There was no control of skin turgor or the appearance of the tongue. The doctor was more interested in sticking to the Swedish Social

Insurance Agencies criteria than me as a human being. The doctor prescribed Zopiclone for my sleep problems and suggested some form of antidepressant. Was the doctor aware that these medicines would weaken my energy field even further? I got the feeling of being declared over imaginative.

How do you tell modern healthcare that you are exposed to black magic? That I have intrusion of negative energy substances on me, that distorted my perception, my emotional life and that exposed my body and brain to negative stress. A black magician who has dedicated her life to controlling my energies, blocking my life force and my flow of life and also sucking energies from me at a distance. A parasitic activity, an energy vampire that took my power.

You hear yourself. It is a completely impossible task. Healthcare is not ready. And if you do not want to be classified as mentally ill, you will have to find ways to explain your precarious situation that has arisen, in other terms to get the sick leave you need. Fatigue was the diagnosis.

The homeostasis made me drawn to the old familiar. It was a catch-22 where I had to remove entities and implants time and time again and realized that it was something that was not aligned with me. I felt helpless and skinless. It was Harry Potter for real. Now I was aware of the attacks. I saw them coming and fought for my life without having the right tools to stop the entities from penetrating my body and distorting my mind. My unconscious allowed it without me being able to consciously end it. It did not help to close the door because everything was happening on an astral plane. I stumbled upon a training in astral self-defense. My self-confidence had hit rock bottom, my self-worth equal to zero and my belief in my own ability non-existent.

The stress I had been unconsciously exposed to for many years had turned my brain into a tough lubrication. I was totally unable to stay focused. My thoughts were like rabbits on a green meadow, I scanned my surroundings and myself to the absurd.

Slowly I realized I could not fix this on my own. I hired a personal coach and also a medium who with impressive precision guided me on the right track. She made me realize the madness in the brooding that was going on in my head and that I have a choice. I decide over my thoughts and my life. By changing my whole thought pattern, I put a stop to the inputs used by the negative energy attacks. If I want to get out of this, it was just a matter of deciding to do so. I understood the seriousness. It was up to me. No one else would fix this for me.

I have realized that I can no longer push back what I experienced during my years as a professional nurse. All the possibilities with this fantastic profession have long since faded and there is only a bad taste left in the mouth. I have been about to leave the profession several times. The idea that a pill should remove all pain and anxiety is also an imaginary world that these companies want us to blindly believe in. These companies allude to our convenience and disregard our own responsibility. We as healthcare professionals are often unconsciously involved in what goes on behind the scenes. The system also does not allow you to look up to get a helicopter perspective. I reacted strongly to all these side effects that come in the way of pharmaceutical drugs. They are not questioned. There are also countless articles about the unhealthy relationship between the pharmaceutical industry and corrupt doctors without results. Big Pharma can control freely with the motto: Money can buy anything. Patient dependence and trust benefit the entire operation. Society has nurtured obedient citizens who put all their trust in a system cluttered with completely unscrupulous creatures. Patients want to believe what the doctor says, even if it echoes contradictory.

It is as if large sections of the population are exposed to mind control. A programming where they repeat their mantra against better knowledge and common sense. Despite the obvious side effects of pharmaceutical drugs, not to mention the highly topical vaccine and its side effects that are now starting to show. Nobody wants to listen and it is prevacated as crazy conspiracy theories. That it would be a conscious system to keep us sick sounds like pure paranoia. Who benefits from it? When did we begin to doubt our own immune system? Common sense is absent in an increasingly bizarre reality.

When the blockages to the Higher Self were removed, my life was turned upside down. It is the human right of every human being to have access to his/her intuition. Everything else is a gross violation of personal integrity. It was this contact with the Higher Self that they blocked me from through black magic. My self-love, my core power and my inner wisdom. I want you to deeply try to imagine what it is they are depriving selected people of. However, it is absolutely necessary for us to control our own energy. If we do not, we give it away to someone else or something else, but when you refuse to give up during difficult circumstances, you are stronger than your destiny.

Those who practice black magic have been seduced and misled by demonic energies and once connected, it is difficult to quit. They steal a little more power and material success at the expense of someone else's life and health and their driving force is jealousy.

LOTTA ASSARSDOTTER

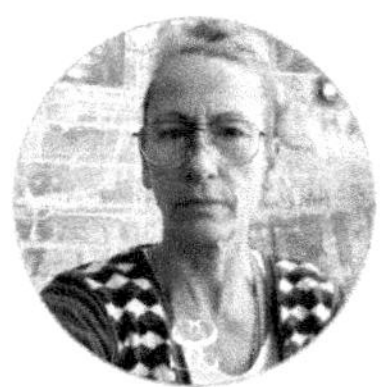

Lotta Assarsdotter paves the way for the care model of the future. Her personal experiences of spiritual abuse as well as what she saw as a professional nurse have left deep traces within her. It took her years to find the right forum to identify the problems.

She no longer believes in the current, modern healthcare system. As an indigo soul, she has the ability to see both sides of the coin. Her findings became the starting point for pioneering online education. Indigos are changing the world and her passion is to make people see what is not visible at first glance, but has a negative effect.

Lotta's unique and personal coaching method is a result of all her experiences. Her personal

journey, from the deepest darkness to where she is today, confirms that it is possible for everyone to successfully make the same journey.

https://linktr.ee/Assarsdotter

12

JOIN ME ON MY JOURNEY TO FINDING IT

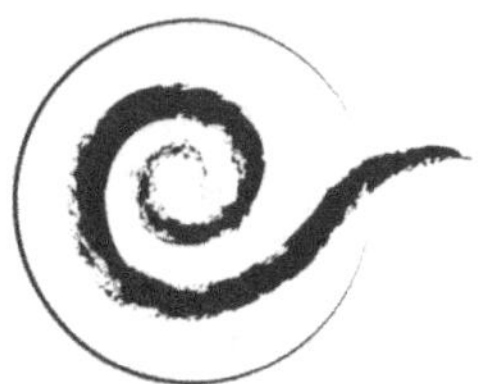

When I close my eyes, I end up in the living room of my childhood home. I lived there with my one year older sister and my mother. We stayed with dad every other weekend. My sister was expressive, dared everything, took to herself and sang like a goddess. I felt insecure and lost, yet filled with love. She was the beautiful swan and I was the little grey duckling.

I looked up to her like no one else. Something I clearly remember was her facial expression when she stood in front of the mirror and sang with her freestyle and headphones in her ears. Not a tone out of tune. I soared slightly away, when I looked at her I dreamed that I was standing next to her. That we sang together. I remember the knot in my stomach as I dreamed of daring. What if I could too? If I ever could, I would never dare.

I grew up in a musical family where my dad played in a dance band. Mom also sang when we were really young. When I was about three years old, mom and dad went their separate ways. We mostly lived with mom, but we were together with dad some weekends.

My father often played in nursing homes where my sister and I would sing some songs. I always stayed in the background. Mostly pretending to sing. My sister sang for both of us. I always thought it was fun to come along but did not really want to sing. It was as if something was stuck in my throat. I had a strong resistance and a choking sensation. I was an insecure and rather shy girl in public. Seen as different by others, I was the squinty idiot. I did not like meeting new people as no one could meet my gaze without becoming as insecure as I was. I felt different and very bluntly stared at. It hit my stomach every time. I never got used to it and would rather always be in my own world. Soared away as soon as I got the chance. In my dreams I was enough, there were no goals that I could ever achieve. I got to be myself. I always knew deep down that I could do and be so much more. If I only got the chance. But who would give me the chance? I realized that I was the only one who could create my own reality. This insight along with a clear goal changed my whole world. I knew it would take a lot of blood, sweat and tears to get there.

When I gave birth to my second child, something happened inside of me that was difficult to put my finger on. I started deeply searching for something and I wanted to work even more thoroughly with myself. I have in a strange way always been close to my intuition but did not know how to listen to it and trust it. I started meditating. Another world opened up for me and I began to see things from a completely different perspective. I received guidance in everything I did and I felt confident that I had a spiritual team behind me that knew how to take the next step. I felt a huge hunger to get ahead, so I searched and searched.

Since I always have had a hard time saying no, I have done everything to make others happy and like me. I knew deep down that it was crazily wrong. You know the feeling in your stomach when you say yes even though you mean no? Your stomach tightens and the anxiety creeps in. Getting to know yourself and your feelings is not easy. You know the difference when you say YES to yourself. The whole existence ends up in harmony. You get relieved. When you are weak and do not have the strength to resist, you accuse yourself of not daring to stand up for the most important person in life!

As I began to say yes to myself, it became more difficult to be in collaborations where you were not sincere. Not being true to oneself is one thing, but not being true to your surroundings is another. I became allergic to fake people who stabbed their loved ones in the back as soon as they were not there. It felt like I ended up in these situations to learn. I automatically started standing up for people who could not defend themselves and the person who started or initiated the drama got offended. This, in turn, of course created problems. I often got into trouble and it was said that I was the one who created the misery. True, but so uncomfortable. Working with oneself is anything but comfortable but a must to get ahead.

One summer morning I sat down with my five-year-old boy on the jetty by the nearby river Dalälven. I drank my coffee and scratched my legs hard. The mosquitoes had bitten me the night before and I can admit that I hate mosquitoes. They're driving me crazy.

My son looks at me, frowns and says: - Mom. You have to make friends with the mosquitoes. Friends do not bite you.

He's so smart. I have such a hard time feeling love for someone who gives me bruises all over my legs.

I often end up in old patterns. My guiding stars show me the way. I have to rethink.

I worked in the travel industry during my first ten years of work. I was brought up well in customer service and I was so confident. Yes, I was a security junkie with a constant need of validation. I knew I did not want to book trips my whole life. I wanted to become something more. I started my own business while working at the travel agency. My husband and I had a hobby where we sawed out wooden hearts and other crafts. I painted and texted on the signs. It became very popular but I realized that it would not last in the long run. Crafts take an enormous amount of time and I put my whole soul into it. I found the joy of creation and that was where I found my energy.

One thing led to the other and I started creating digitally. It took more of my time and I disappeared into my world of creativity. At the same time, my sister's husband started a web agency with his cousin. I thought it was so exciting, but knew nothing about the web. I started practicing. I felt this immense joy in everything I did that is hard to explain. But you know that feeling of tingling in the stomach? When you have tried and tried and then succeeded with something that has been difficult. In the beginning, I had a hard time dealing with my ups and downs. When I succeeded, I became so happy that I knew neither out nor in. When I failed, my whole world collapsed. So much emotion, so much of everything.

A few years ago I made a decision and created. I had a clear goal of what I wanted in my life. To be able to work with what I love. But it felt so far away. My workplace was in a phase of change and we agreed that I would leave. It was time. Troublesome thoughts kept coming up about how I was going to cope. How do I get a job? Can you work with your hobby? The security junkie in me was terrified. The thoughts of disaster and the rush of happiness took turns.

I've always said I'm not a salesperson. Just panicked at the thought. Many tried to say that I must begin to dare to pick up the phone and tell people about what I do.

One of my closest friends has been a great support in my journey when it comes to empowering me to start being brave. He worked as a manager in another place and invited me there so that I could get started and meet customers. Once there, it turned out after a few days that I had to take the first step myself. I was so nervous before the trip so I was shaking just thinking about it. I was sitting in the hotel room. It was quiet and sad. He worked long days and we ate dinner together. During dinner, he tells me the purpose of why I have to take the plunge. He made me dare to leave home because there I had no one to distract me. I had to slowly go into myself and realize what I needed to do. I understood the purpose but was not so happy that I now have to dare. Thought it was enough outside the box to get there. The next day I sat down and made a presentation. I remember how I was shaking when I dialed the number on my cell phone to call the first company. It turned out to be easier than I thought and I made a few subsequent calls. I dared more and more and stopped shaking after the third call.

In the beginning, when I had customer meetings, I was so nervous that I felt bad. Do not know how many times I have thought about why I exposed myself to it.

The more self-esteem I gained, the more changes I began to experience. Each new customer I would meet, I always sat down for a while before and reflected. I saw colors and a lot of other things that spun like a wheel of fortune before my eyes.. I felt with curiosity who the person was who would soon step through the door. I was not nervous anymore. It was a wonderful feeling, to be able to stand in my power. To meet people who want my help to find their IT. I go through my working days with euphoria, adrenaline rush, happiness, an endless creativity and very often also with frustration, a patience that sways, blood and, sweat and tears. I really love it!

It has been a hard journey to find myself but wow how nice it feels not to be limited in life. My brain is now connected to my heart and my stomach. When you do something you love, there are no limits. When I am in my creative power, I am at home. There are no worries, no drama, no stress.

I build my customer relationships on trust, and continuous dialogue. High in spirit and good communication are a must for us to be able to create magic together. I believe that if you can think it, you can create it. I find the solutions to my customers' IT requests through intuition and feeling.

I really do not like to say that you should find yourself. What I have seen during my years is that you can create yourself. The creative power is enormous and infinite. If only you dare.

In order for my brain to be in total relaxation, the best way for me is to be creative and to create. One evening it became a kind of 3D staircase. A staircase can be interpreted in two ways. You can climb to reach your goals. But you can also descend yourself down. This is definitely not a negative thing. On the contrary; You walk outside your comfort zone and develop on the way down.

When you find time for reflection, the best ideas and the funniest future plans usually come. I have a clear goal, but often doubt my own ability to go that far. I'm so happy about all the amazing people I have in my network. They push me and press those little magic buttons that make it worthwhile to continue fighting for what I dream of.

Like the Swedish saying - we will go all in and then increase!

But increasing and not realizing when it's time to pull the brakes is something I have a hard time regulating. I went for too long in the wrong vibration and crashed. Three years ago, when I was at my peak in growing my business, I began to doubt myself. I was cowardly and took a job with a friend because I thought I could work twice as much for a while.

I totally went against my will and dream. It was a failure. Six months later, I did not get out of bed. I had been trying for so long. I felt no joy in life. I had no energy left. My life energy had been swallowed up by my inability to listen inwardly.

I started meditating and all of a sudden I experienced my feelings more easily. I closed my eyes and saw myself standing there on the mountain. When I looked up I saw the crack and a precipice. I had two choices. Either stay in fear or dare to jump over to the side that makes me whole. I chose to jump. Without parachute and lifeline. I did it!

But not without all the cheers from my loved ones. They are and have been absolutely fantastic during all the ups and downs.

The only time I was anxiety free was when I got to go into digital creation. I was swallowed up by the screen and I found my healing in the pen. In this way, I went into the cellular level in different graphic techniques and I never gave up until I succeeded.

Slowly but surely I began to smile at the world again. I was free. I could feel joy in a new way. I was born again and I started to expand. Acquired my very first own office in a beautiful manor, decorated with tenderness and a huge happiness. Every day as I stepped into the office, I looked around. Pinch me!

Once I decided never to go against the gut feeling again, things started to happen. As soon as I finished a project, the next one presented itself. I felt grateful that my reality had become the one I could only dream of.

I realized for the first time in my life that I'm good at something. Now I understand what my sister's secret was. She sang more than she talked. She practiced, practiced and practiced. So similar but still so different. I have found my true art form – digital design.

When doubt once again entered my life, so did Mira. She came in with great visions and a mindset I have never seen in my life. She has been through all levels of hell in her life and still stands up. Smiling. Loving. Pushing others forward. She saw me and gave me the missing pieces of how to control my energy field and vibration. She stands strong and does not care if I am at my worst or at my best.

Now I can manage the constant ebb and flow of life, energies and feelings. I have come to love the down as much as the ups, because it is that motion that creates the flow forward. None of my emotions, thoughts or expressions are wrong. I am strong. I am fine.

I am surrounded by people who share the same view of what life is meant to be. We do not always share the same goals or dreams, but our vibration and energy are definitely at the same level and I do not have to consider if I am good enough or not. I am fully allowed to be me and I am fully committed to keeping this attitude in life.

I am surrounded by people who support me, even though they do not understand my dreams or see them as doable as I do. I am allowed to be wrong and end up right. For the first time in life I feel that I am worthy both at my worst and at my best. Laughter and joy surrounds me, tears are shared. Those moments when anxiety comes knocking I am in control and I am allowed to express it without fear of being judged as weak.

Mira always reminds me of the great wisdom of Mother Pinetree: All emotions are allowed. They do not control our actions, unless we let them. Emotions guide us in life and keep us on the right track. Emotions are tools in life and when I use them right, I cannot go wrong. I am allowed.

MARLENE MÅRTENS ASPGREN

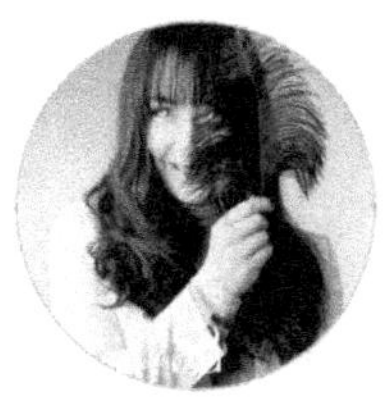

Marlene Mårtens Aspgren is an intuitive web designer, marketer and graphic designer. She is CEO of a web and marketing agency. She is also Marketing And Sales Manager at the Tourist Attraction Visit Abisko in Lapland.

With color, form, and an enormous commitment, she creates magic together with her customers. She builds her customer relationships on trust, and continuous dialogue. High in spirit and with good communication she is able to create digital magic. She believes that if you can dream it, you can create it. She finds people's IT solutions by being intuitive, steadfast, humble, enormously creative by using her magical fingertip feeling.

She created her own reality through her creativity and now lives her dream with all her heart and soul. She dares to challenge by making full use of her strong intuition to arouse the customers' desire to expand, both in themselves as well as in their business.

Website: www.maartens.se
Email: marlene@maartens.se
Facebook: www.facebook.com/Maartens.se
Instagram: www.instagram.com/maartens_design
LinkedIn: www.linkedin.com/in/marlene-mårtens-aspgren
Linktr.ee: www.linktr.ee/marlenemartensaspgren

13

THE MAGPIE MAGIC

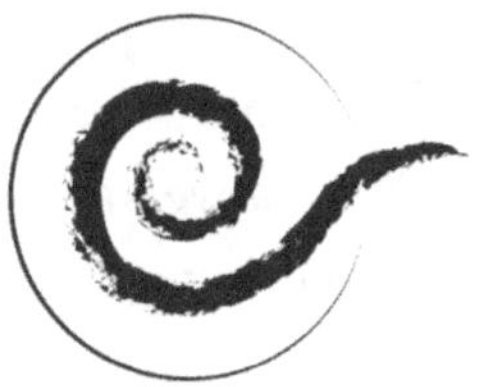

Before we start, remember this.

I love my Mother and when she leaves this linear time and space she shall be free from guilt and regret. She will leave loved and honoured as the Mother she is. She will stand with our ancestors.

Strong. Proud. Wise.

With no wounds in her soul.

"The Magpie does not weave the magical threads of life, but she reads them well. She knows all the knots and flaws by heart, since she observes. She watches and learns, she creates the balance where none is found. She combines the God and the Goddess. The light and the dark. The good and the bad. She does that 'cause she can travel within the threads of life and combine them all. She creates beauty wherever she goes, this is why it is said she loves all that shines. She harvests the power of beauty and hands it to those in need. The Magpie Magic tears illusions apart 'cause beauty lies in truth. The Magpie Magic sets all in motion 'cause it makes the weak threads strong."

The song, is what I grew up hearing. Not until adulthood did I understand that it was a teaching, not a child's song. My grandmother sang it to me. Year after year I heard these words never knowing she was singing about me. The Magpie and her magic.

Where does a story begin? I could say that this story started with my great great great grandmother who foretold my birth. But, this story starts with where I am today. Who I am today. I fully accepted my role in this linear time and space reality, but I have also come to terms with the fact that circular time has no beginning nor an end. It is constantly flowing and impossible to measure due to its magical nature. I will tell you more about the magic of the circular time in the forthcoming book Multiverse, so there is no need for us to consider time as we travel through the Threads of Life creating me.

In the darkest of dark, you shall find your light,
your power and your true calling.

She left me, my mother. There lying on the bed. Alone. Abandoned. Not wanted. No one knows for how long, but there was still enough life in me to stand here and now alive and well.

Breathing gratefully and proud of who I am and knowing in my heart that this is the right moment in this linear time and space reality to let this go. It humbled me, it gave me wisdom beyond what any school could give. It has given me the power to forgive and to understand that power in action. Forgiveness can create wonderful things if you have the courage to practise it from the bottom of your heart.

I was told this story many times as a child. Your mother couldn't take care of you. She left you. She chose the partying. She couldn't handle responsibility. She was selfish.

I wanted to see for myself what made her decide to leave me alone on that bed for days. I have asked her, but she cannot remember, or she doesn't want to remember. Either way, she couldn't give an answer.

I lay my trust in my practise and in the Wisdom of Mother Pinetree. In the ceremony I travelled in the primordial vibration of the drum and sought to see that day, that moment, when my mother decided to abandon me. I went back to face that moment of fear with the mindset of changing the energy to fearless and fierce instead of fear.

Instead I found myself seeing my mother in that moment broken. No hope and full of sadness. She was afraid, ashamed, in pain, lost and completely alone. I had a choice to make, to use the power of anger to cut the cord and walk away. Use the energy to make me fearless and fierce. Or, I could do something that would unleash all the love she actually felt for me. At this moment I embraced her with all my love, forgiveness and power and with all the love in my heart and whispered in her ear. "I will be OK and you will love me and be proud of me. Do what you need to do, to survive. I see you. I forgive you."

A few days went by and my mother came to see me. She told me that she had dreamt the strangest dream. She had seen me as a baby on a bed, so full of light that she was blinded by it. She had closed her eyes and when she opened them I was gone. The bed was empty. She also told me that someone had whispered to her in that dream that she was forgiven. She had woken up and felt light, as a burden had been lifted from her shoulders and as if it was ok to be without guilt.

This is the Magpie Magic I possess. I untied a knot in one of the threads in the Web of Life and therefore lifted the guilt from my mother. I took a loose end of the thread and connected it to me tightly. Straight into my heart.

"When life hurts you.
You need to love it back."
~Mira Hilaria Mård~

I grew up in my grandmother's care. Then I moved back home to my mother and father. They had made a new start in a new country. Happy at first, then it all turned upside down. I grew up in violence and I did not want to live in the real world. I found my escape in the small woods surrounding the suburb I grew up in. In these woods I created a magical world of my own, seeking console from the inhabitants of the forest. Since I was born with the ability to see the elves and the trolls, I had company at all times.

I survived by living in two worlds: the world of spirit and the world as we know it. Fully aware of the difference between them.

As a child I had dreams. When I turned 14 those dreams were torn apart. Brutally and with no warning they were taken. Shattered and broken, just as my heart and soul would be for a long time. I was raped. Abused and burned. Literally burned. I still carry the scars on my body as a reminder. Now those scars are covered by tattoos as a manifestation of the fact that I have the power to rewrite the story by mending the broken threads in the Web of Life.

I was forced into silence. It was covered up. No drama, no trial. Nothing but silence and I accepted that silence as the good obedient girl I was. Accepting this illusion made me accept a lot in the future. This is where I accepted the illusion of my unworthiness. I played this part well.

I was abused. I abused me. I allowed others to abuse me. I suffocated myself and my Magpie Magic. Tightly closing my eyes, silencing my tongue and paralysing my soul. I was pretending to be alive and well, but as Magpie Magic tears illusions apart the play along life crumbled to pieces again and again. The illusion surrounding me was bound to break. But it broke me first.

If you cannot embrace what has been, you cannot be in the now, nor become what you are meant to be. This insight hit me hard, but it also defined me. This meant that I had to set myself free from the chains of the past. Some of those chains were created by people that I couldn't reach out to. Either because I didn't want to or because of the fact that they are no longer among us. But the magic of the Magpie Magic is just that – I don't have to reach out. I simply travel the threads on the Web of Life and get closure. Those of spirit I am able to reach out to, but I didn't feel the need to hear apologies from them. I wanted definite closure from my part, in my process, for me.

The hardships of life humbled me and opened my heart to the wisdom of the ancient ones. Of this I am certain. And I rest well in this insight of myself. I am fully aware of the fact that I could have made a career as a lawyer, but I am grateful that I chose the path of my ancestral mothers and their wisdom. It gives me joy and it gives me a true connection with me, my ancestors and creation itself. My essence is in balance, rather than in fame or built from bitterness and hate towards those who hurt me as a child. I show people on a daily basis that one can heal oneself. Fully and completely, by simply being true to one's own unique vibration and Path of Life.

The hardships of life also shaped me into the healer I am. I do not have a judgemental bone in my body. Nothing surprises me and no one ever feels shame in front of me. I shiver in front of people leaning on their inner victim and I question the fact that they choose to stay in the vibration of 'victim'. The healing process will only start when you break up with the victim within you and aim for the healing and power of experience. You need to be able to welcome the new you fully, in all its glory and pain. I know that most of us aim for healing without pain, but in order to release it, you need to acknowledge it. This doesn't mean that you need to relive it in any way. Just accept it and acknowledge it.

Being un-chosen made me see the difference between need-based love and pure love. This is why I will never fall into needing again. I don't want to need someone, need changes. I want to live in that constant ebb and flow or love that makes every day count. Pure love has its base in aspects of respect, loyalty, truth and love. Your need doesn't affect all that. Need and greed is what eats you up from the inside, never satisfied, always looking for the better deal. As I explored Magpie Magic, I understood why this vision of love is of importance for me, and you.

Imagine this: you fall in love and you have that first fight. A knot appears on the thread representing your relationship in the Web of Life. If you untie it rapidly, it leaves no mark. If you ignore it, it tightens over time. In order for you to ignore that knot tightening, you start to embrace all the things you need, big or small, they legitimate you ignoring the knot. If you do not need anything but pure love from your partner, this knot cannot be ignored. It will be acknowledged and healed. When this happens, the thread gets stronger and will continue to grow stronger for every knot healed.

Rage tears the threads apart. Flying around in the storms caused by the rage. The threads flying around like this makes you eventually unfocused, rootless and lost.

"The rage begins where ceremony is excluded.
The rage is what closes the doors to beauty, ceremony and obedience.
Obedience is what creates surrender, surrender creates growth."
~Mother Pinetree~

I have carried the vibration of anger for many years. It gave me nothing but grief, an empty feeling of bitterness. By reconnecting with my Magpie Magic, my traditions and the love I carry in my heart I could let go of anger and turn towards a harmonious vibration within me. Letting go of anger does not mean that you sweep away what has happened. What happens is that anger can no longer consume your energy and make your vibration disharmonic. It gives you freedom and healthy boundaries based upon experience rather than emotion.

Sorrow makes the threads heavy, weighing you down. Unattended, they eventually break you down. Stagnation, bitterness and not lifting your eyes beyond what makes you lost.

"Let your heart cry out it's sadness.
Let your heart break into a thousand pieces.
When you mend it, your heart will be stronger and more
beautiful that it has ever been. It will also be wiser than before."
~My grandmother~

It is important to recognize the power of these threads and tend to them. The weak threads will eventually break and when they do, there will be a tear in the Web of Life. That tear may cause great problems for you when meeting new people or opportunities. That tear is what makes you disconnect from your natural, harmonical vibration, which is your guiding star in life. This is Vibrational Healing and differs a lot from the Magpie Magic which is more about the art of seeing, mending and altering the threads that create the Web of Life. Believe it or not, the Web of Life is in constant change. Every moment in your life you actually stand with a thread in your hand and your actions attach it to the Web of Life. Just as easily as the steps you take in life moves you along the Path of Life. All things are connected, the method and descriptions are the only thing that sets them apart.

What happens when we have too many loose ends in our lives?

For starters, we cannot weave new threads and the loose ends (threads) drains our energy and eventually our power and vibration. We lose hope, we lose will, we lose direction and determination. We are no longer steadfast, driven and visionary. We simply fade away and shortly thereafter our dreams fade. We accept the fact that we merely exist to survive life, instead of living it to the fullest.

These loose threads also cause wide open entrances in our energy fields. We become vulnerable and it is easy for the human energy predators to get what they want and need from us. This is why we need to gather those loose ends and create closure. Every loose end tied and closure done, your energy fields come closer to the magic of the circular time and space. The energy fields are strengthened and the flow in your energy field changes into something that reflects rather than absorbs.

Simultaneously you are deepening your understanding of and for situations in the past. You fall into insight and forgiveness. You find new power within you and your original vibration grows stronger and stronger. All of the sudden you realize the beauty of being you.

I never understood why this process surprises us so much – realizing who we are. It should be the most natural thing in our lives to know who we are, what we are meant to do and what magic and beauty we possess. But still, we are surprised by the greatness of it all and I am grateful for each and every time I get to witness this process and healing in the people who seek my Magpie Magic. My heart whispers every time *"this is what you are meant to do"*.

At the same time as I know that this choice was made for me long before I was born, I know that I made it myself as a child and again as an adult. There never were any questions about following this particular Path of Life. I always say "life means me well" even though the days might be too tough to handle.

My essence, my vibration, tells me that this is the only way to go. My heart is true to it and my soul feels satisfied every time I practise the medicine given to me by my ancestral mothers. I am one of many, I am a manifestation of my ancestral mothers. I am the daughter of those mothers who have walked the Path of Life before me. Always guiding my steps towards where I stand today. Always on the frontier in order to give women the freedom of practising our magical medicine from within again without being tortured or burned.

My mission in this linear time and space reality is to show every woman sharing my Path of Life with me for a period of time how to connect with their vibration, master it, heal with it and find their own version of Magpie Magic.

Yes, dear.
You have it too.
Within you.

MIRA HILARIA MÅRD

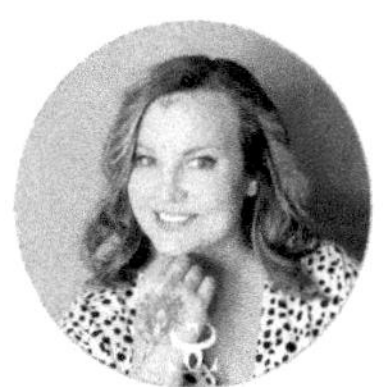

Mira Hilaria Mård is a perspicacious channel for the spirit realm and with her down to earth attitude she is a fierce living artist integrating the Magpie Magic in her everyday life.

She is steadfast in manifesting her vision and an inspiring channel for the Spirit Realm. She is an international bestselling author and her book Wisdom of Mother Pinetree is a revelation of how to integrate your spirituality and shamanic lifestyle into your everyday life.

Her life-like courses and individual sessions are magical and life-changing for those who dare to surrender to the transformative process and fully bloom on the Path of Life.

Mira, unique in her field, raised in a shamanic family and managing a legacy of her ancestral mothers. This makes her authentic and singular in her field. She is also a fierce entrepreneur and CEO of a rapidly growing business with a shamanic leadership.

www.linktr.ee/miramard

14

JUMPING REALMS

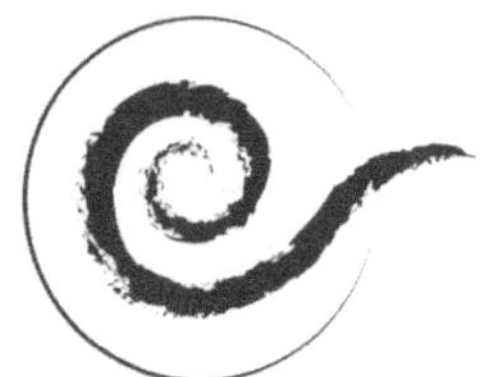

I'm about to tell you something that I've only told two other people. Two people I trusted dearly who may not always understand me but seem to love me anyway. I whispered this truth to them over a glass of wine while we were wrapped in conversation and immersed in the moment and then waited for their reaction. I wondered if they would think I was crazy, but instead they received what I was saying with love and grace and in the truest form of who they are they tried to understand the words I was telling them. I'm asking you to receive this with as much grace and understanding as they did. There are things in this world we can't completely understand but still know are true. You may not understand what I'm about to tell you but please trust that I am only speaking from my truth and explaining things the best way I am capable.

I JUMPED REALMS AND AM NOW LIVING IN A NEW REALITY

5 months ago at the recommendation of a friend I picked up the book (or audio book actually) "Breaking the Habit of Being Yourself" by Dr. Joe Dispenza. I would listen to this book everyday and even though it

was quite deep and much of it was over my head, I consumed and digested as much of it as possible. The key to this book though is not in reading or even understanding the content, the key to this book is implementing the practices and exercises—consistently. Literally breaking the habit of being yourself by letting go of the smaller parts, habits and conditioning that keep you stuck in one paradigm while welcoming the highest and best version of yourself (otherwise known as manifesting your best life.)

Everyday I would do the meditations and everyday I would find myself acting less like a victim which was one habit I was desperate to let go of. That and being less negative, which goes hand and hand with that victim mentality doesn't it? Online and to my friends I put on a cheery disposition and the ultimate positive outlook, but in the darkness that creeps inside my head and out loud to my now ex-partner who was my current partner at the time, I would seep down the spirals of sorrow and self pity allowing myself to wallow in uncertainty and mistrust for what was and could be possible. It really is a terrible existence to reside in and if you're someone who comes to this place frequently, I promise there are much better places for you to live. Regardless though, if you find yourself feeling sorry for yourself, have angry outbursts, indulging in procrastination that keeps you stuck or partake in any other negative behaviours consistently and believe they may be a reason you're not moving forward, I strongly recommend this book and in doing the exercises and most importantly... the meditations. "Breaking the Habit of Being Yourself" by Dr. Joe Dispenza.

I was doing the daily meditations and recognizing things were changing in my own behaviors but things hadn't really shifted in terms of my outward reality yet, but they were about to.

I was exclusively working for women in the publishing industry in my virtual assistant business at the time. Supporting small female owned publishing houses who were producing multi-author books. I had been doing this work for some time and decided I was ready to take my love for words, story, connection and ultimate self-expression do a major upleving in my business and start my own publishing company. I invested in a high dollar mentorship with a woman who would help me become successful in this endeavor. I took a deep breath and dove straight in. I kept meditating, I kept practicing letting go and I kept leaning into my higher self.

Two weeks later I stood nose to nose with my husband of 18 years and partner of 24 years as he told me he wasn't happy in our marriage. He rattled off all the reasons he wanted to leave as he packed a bag and walked out the door. I was gutted. I sat in this mounting pile of uncertainty and despair and wondered why this was happening to me and why now at such a delicate time in my business and career.

I kept doing the meditations. I kept leaning into letting go. I kept trusting that I was shredding what was holding me back, which I was. But I hadn't realized yet that my marriage was one of the things I needed to let go of in order to start living the life I was envisioning.

THE TRIP

I was working at home and the walls were closing in on me. I couldn't escape the grief and the burden of responsibilities I was facing. Summer was quickly approaching and the kids would be home from school soon. I needed to arrange for their care, entertainment, nourishment, as well as also being the primary one helping them to process the emotional toll the separation was having.

It felt like too much.

That's when I had the thought of taking a trip. For years I had wanted to take an extended working vacation but my husband's schedule never allowed for it. With that out of the way, I thought this is the perfect time to make it happen. So I did. I scoured the internet for long term vacation rentals within my budget. I wanted something on the water. I wanted to wake up everyday and feel like I was in paradise. I narrowed down my selection to a couple potential properties and ended up settling on one beautiful lake front cottage in Bainbridge Georgia. Bainbridge Georgia has a population of about 12,000 people just west of Alabama - a 45 minute drive south and you're in Tallahassee Fl. I didn't know why I picked this place or even more likely why this place summoned me to it but I believe I understand now.

IT WASN'T PARADISE, IT WAS A SWAMP

Or at least that's what it felt like when we arrived at 8:00 at night and it was getting dark. I had messed up the dates for the reservation and was having to negotiate an early arrival with the owner. He was making it work but we wouldn't be able to check in until 9:00. This was the second day of driving 13 hours and we were so ready to get settled in but instead we had to wait for the cleaning lady to finish. As I drove to the property I kept looking for the lake. This place is directly on Lake Seminole, so where is the lake? All I could see was trees. Massive trees lining the road for as far as the eye could see. I located the property and stepped outside to nature's orchestra.The loud humm of crickets, frogs, toads, birds and other critters made this rural Georgia town feel creepy. The lady cleaning the house stepped outside and I asked her "What is that sound?" she stopped and listened for a minute before replying "that's just normal." The vibrant sounds were not something I was used to hearing in Colorado and it was a bit unsettling at first. I walked around to the back of the house to where the lake was. The lake was covered in mossy grass and at first glance looked like a swamp.

When we finally made our way inside it was a hodgepodge little house, clean but kind of funky. This backwoods lake house with nature screaming at me located directly on a swampy lake made me feel like I had been dropped right into a scene from the movie Deliverance. I went to bed with an uneasy feeling wondering if I had made the right choice in bringing us all this way and woke up turning straight to my journal to process what I was experiencing. With my journal and pen in hand I started to write and channel guidance. "What am I supposed to experience on this trip?" I asked "we wouldn't have brought you all this way by accident, it was on purpose. Hidden gems EVERYWHERE Things aren't as they appear. That nervousness in your stomach is asking for you to surrender to things as they are and not what you plan for them to be. Please listen closely and observe nature that's all around you - it is your teacher." And so I did.

NATURE SPEAKS

We had a poor WIFI signal at the house we were staying in, making it difficult to work. We were on the outskirts of Baindbridge at least a 30 minute drive to get to a public place where I could connect to WIFI. Looking back now, I see it as a blessing. It created the quiet disconnect that I truly needed and an invitation to be outside. Everyday I would sit outside on the dock of that lake in this little echo system that made up the most unique place I have ever visited. I listened to the singing birds, the croaking frogs and chirping crickets and begged the lake to tell me why I was there. To reveal to me the lesson I had come all this way for. There wasn't anything obvious about it other than the perfectness of it all. The lush green grass, the quietness beyond the hum of nature, the daily rain storms that would cool things off just enough, the hues of pinks and orange that painted the sky at sunset or the crane that would visit every morning. Yes, all of this is so perfect, nature is perfect in so many ways but what does that have to do with me and how does this help me move beyond the grief and rejection of my marriage ending or the uncertainty that lies ahead?

Our trip consisted of frequent visits to Panama City Beach, a few excursions to second hand stores, local attractions and lots of sitting in our very own nature preserve right there on Lake Seminole. Nature's impression imprinted on me during that trip changed me to my core. I underappreciated its glory while I was there and now I find myself missing the vibrant aliveness that can only be experienced in a place like that. I hope to return there someday for a second dose of learning from the magnificent mother earth in all her glory. This time, I promise to not miss a single moment of it by second guessing or wondering if I'm in the right place. I'll know that I am right where I need to be and it will feel much more like home to me.

The secret of my visit wouldn't be revealed to me until months later when I realized how connected I had become to mother nature. Mother earth was speaking to me through the flowers, trees, rocks, water and soil. I started to hear the vibration and unique expressions and messages about our existence would become revealed when I asked her for wisdom.

We returned from our trip and I found myself getting sucked back into the sadness of my current circumstances. Even though I felt refreshed and something new inside me felt awake for the first time in a long time, the ending of an 18 year old marriage is something you must grieve along with processing the slew of other things that come up during such transition.

The difference though is how I allowed myself to process these emotions. I stopped labeling them good or bad but instead just allowed them to be. I sat with them and in them for as long as they needed to linger and allowed them to pass through when they were ready. I don't rush these feelings, instead I lean into experiencing them fully, getting swallowed in the grief, caught up in the excitement or enraged with the anger. I don't want to dull any of it. Just like nature works in complete unison, so do our feelings and emotions when we allow them to be.

JUMPING REALMS

Circling back around to the point of this story. Sharing about the trip to Lake Seminole was a bit of a detour but such an important part of my healing, letting go, expansion and learning how to dance in the storm.

The hard truth that I came here to share is that even though my husband initiated our divorce, I have since realized and believe that by practicing those daily meditations and letting go of the smaller parts of myself to make room for my higher self to manifest is when I jumped realms into a new reality. Leaving the life I had built behind. My ex-husband is happy in that other realm, he didn't want to come with me. So now I find myself in this brand new realm, where everything looks the same but NOTHING is. Just like my guides shared with me when I asked them for guidance on our trip, "NOTHING is as it seems." I had to come to terms with this reality. That I was the one who actually left. That in some metaphysical or spiritual realm I made this conscious decision, I aligned my energy in just the right way to open a portal to a different realm of existence and when the time was right - I jumped. So here I am, the same person but also very different. With many of the same people in my life but experiencing very different relationships with them. I even changed my name from Nikki to Nicolette (my birth name) and am living a totally different life now.

This story might sound crazy to you or maybe you'll hear my story and think "Life changes, that doesn't mean you're living in a new reality." Which may very well be true. It's not how things appear on the outside but how things feel in the deepest parts of me that brought me to this realization.

A blossoming publishing company, new and old friends coming out of the woodwork to support me, to see me and honor my purpose and unique essence—the type of unconditional support I have only longed for. Or maybe it's the earth angels showing up in the most remarkable ways, helping and guiding me through this transition, reminding me of how I am always supported. Or maybe it's my ability to manifest things so easily.

All of this could be just a personal expansion and transformation. It could be me seeing the bright side of a personal tragedy or trying to claim more control from what once felt like a lopsided and powerless life event but it also could be exactly what I am telling you. For years I felt stuck in an old paradigm where people didn't really understand me and therefore couldn't fully support me. A paradigm I could only gain so much traction in before hitting a brick wall. A place I was slowly but certainly losing myself to and was experiencing the smothering of my heart and soul and then all of a sudden I feel more like me than I have in years. A braver, more confident and fuller me.Unapologetic in my ability to share more of my truth with the world. The moment my husband left I gave myself permission to play full out, to not hold back or try to fit into someone else's expectations of what I should be. I am now on a mission, a soul mission that I believe is the reason I am here on earth. To encourage and explore total and complete self-expression of the heart and soul for me, my clients and the world. By sharing more of ourselves with the world, our tragedies and triumphs, struggles and breakthroughs and how we have experienced all of it will make the world a much more understanding and compassionate place.

NICOLETTE HALLADAY

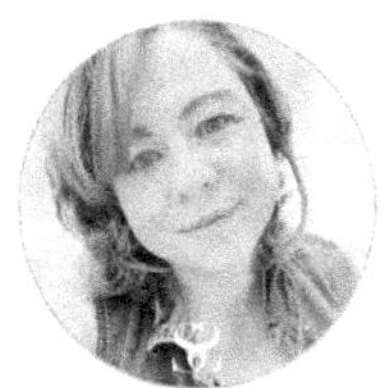

Nicolette Halladay is the founder of Inspired Hearts Publishing—an independently owned publishing house focused on multi-author book collaborations, created to share the unconventional and heartfelt stories of entrepreneurs. Giving business owners a platform to tell their stories, own their talents, and leverage their personal story to grow their business.

She started her entrepreneurial journey by launching a virtual assistant agency where she learned the fundamentals of online business and found her love for publishing through niching down in her business and exclusively supporting other female-owned publishers in the backend of their business until she took the leap to branch out starting her own publishing company.

Nicolette does the work she does because of the time, financial and creative freedoms offered in entrepreneurship and her love for this work that pushes her to explore and express total and complete self-expression of the heart and soul for herself and her clients.

https://linktr.ee/Nicolette111

15

SIERRA'S STORY

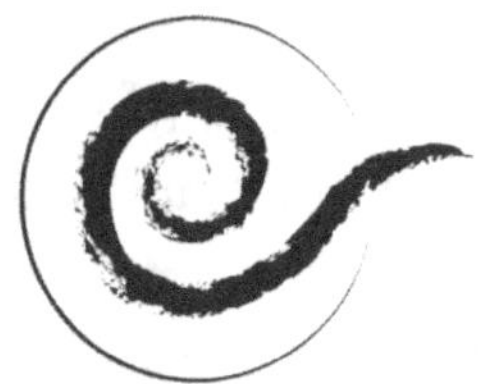

By owning our story we can fundamentally change more than just ourselves; we can change the world.

We never know who we're going to become, much less what it's going to take to get us there. We each have a story. We each have a storm. Very rarely during the storm, can we appreciate who it's making us become.

There are the storms that happen to us, well beyond our control. But there is yet another kind of storm; my most important storms are the storms that I made myself.

Now on the other side, I view storms, every storm, as an invitation. It's an invitation to who we can become.

The most powerful stories we tell, are to ourselves

For so long the stories I told myself about who I was growing up, about my childhood, about the core truths of me, were wrong.

I sat on the floor of the home I was born in. My young daughter played next to me. I had three days to go through everything I owned. Give it away, burn it, or fit it into the two boxes that I could take with me. In front of me, in boxes, were journals from high school and every photograph I'd ever taken before life could fit on a microchip. Every letter from all of my dead grandparents, dear friends, early childhood mementos: first drawings, and stuffed animals. My life, in its physical record, cluttered the floor. I was flooded with memories of all that I had been.

But as I read these letters, as I read my own horrific handwriting, as I tore the pages in my journal that I stapled together so no one would ever read them, I was presented with a very different version of myself than the one I had been carrying around in my mind.

I read letters from boys that had loved me. I thought those letters were proof, confirming an impenetrable story I had crafted that I was unloved, unlovable. My response to childhood sexual trauma, maybe. But right there on the page, as clear as day was the love I had somehow missed at the time. There hadn't been room in my story for their love.

Sitting there, 30 years later, juxtaposed with these letters, was proof of what I was longing for, right in front of me. One of my core beliefs, that no one had ever loved me, was shattered by a crumpled old piece of paper. But I wasn't done. There was a lot more to read and a lot more to burn.

Reading my shitty high school poetry, I found beautiful, insightful literary gems in my own scrawl. Another core belief was challenged. The story shaped by growing up dyslexic, was that I couldn't be a writer. I was blind to the fact that I have been writing for nearly 30 years. The story was the only thing holding me back.

Flannery O'Connor wrote, "I write to discover what I know." In the reading of my own words, a primary source analysis of who I was, disproved, who I *thought* I was. After reading and burning most of my life treasures, storing a few random things that I could not bear to part with, I walked away from the boxes of my life.

I walked away, having to reconsider who I was on every level. If I had gotten this much so wrong, where else was my story fundamentally built on lies and full of bullshit? It was terrifying, and yet, so incredibly liberating, and energizing to discover a new interpretation of myself.

What else was not correct? What an exciting question.

HOW WRITING CHANGED ME:

I didn't know my truth until I wrote it. Writing for me is revelatory.

What if the seeds of our next adventure are ready, planted, and sprouting even while we are in the midst of our winter, our crises, our falling apart?

There's a tree I walk by every day. Today, it's losing half of its leaves. Meanwhile, it's in full bloom, putting out flowers and new leaves.

Having grown up in the Northeast of the United States, this tree seems to defy nature as I understood it with its distinct seasons: winter, spring, summer, fall. One thing had to end, and die, before another thing could start and bloom.

Now, having lived 13 years in Colombia, South America, the trees here are teaching me another way. What if we don't have to distinguish between one thing ending and another thing beginning. The sprouts, life, the fuel of our next iteration, are already in play, are already well established in the unraveling and the falling apart.

Since being here I have learned to see the seeds in the midst of the destruction, that to me, tempers that perspective, the storm itself. When I see new growth, in the wintertime, the bleak, dreary seemingly endless winter does not seem so bad. So this is my story.

My storm. My storm was largely self-inflicted because I couldn't see the life at the end of the tunnel. I couldn't see how the struggle was teaching me yet, my storm was exactly the lesson I needed to get where I am. The obstacles, at this moment, are exactly what I need to get me where I'm going. In my life so far, I have reinvented multiple times: changing careers, living in foreign countries, moving from the USA to China to Colombia, being a high school teacher, a yoga studio owner, a single mother, an author, women's empowerment leader, and running an all-female publishing company. Now, I am seeing how all of my previous iterations were the necessary foundation for my current expression.

Rather than the obstacles and the struggles of our life being the things to avoid, I see them as the things that forge us, make us who we are and show us what we're capable of. Storms challenge us to grow stronger. Or they devastate us. The storms that tested me the most were internal.

Growing up dyslexic, I learned to read when I was 13 and struggled with written communication for years after that. After becoming a teacher in my 20's, I really felt the urge to write. But the story I had about myself, this perception I had crafted, was the primary obstacle. I finally sat down to write my first book in 2006 but years later that unfinished manuscript is still on a hard drive somewhere. That dream withered.

At different times, I returned to my writing nonchalantly blogging, making random posts with no specific intention. I never gave writing my heart because I never believed that I could ever be a writer, so I never tried. Until over 10 years later, after my daughter was born, I felt struck with the urge to write again. The birth process taught me about the incredible gifts on the other side of struggle and pain. Through my adventures with my own limiting story, I began to courageously write - quite badly I might add. But I wrote anyway. This is the part that I think is the most important.

This is the part where the storm winds shifted. When the internal storm of doubt stopped being the loudest voice in my head. I wrote regardless. In the act of doing so, I learned something more important than great grammar and the ins-and-outs of the publishing industry. I learned faith: faith in myself, in my ability to grow into the next thing that I am becoming. When harnessed, that faith will get you through anything.

Reinvention through letting my own internal storm winds quiet, taught me how to let my own path unfold in front of me. Since then, I have written two books on my own: ***How Change Really Happens*** and ***Date Yourself,*** contributed to three other collaborations, plus at the time of this writing I am embarking on a three-part book series called ***Story Ink*** about writing and publishing. I am committed to writing five more collaborations this year. Just a few years ago the idea of publishing my own book seemed an impossibility, and now I have opened a publishing company. *Because of my first publishing opportunity, I am a huge fan of book collaborations, like this one. We offer the same opportunity to get published with us by writing a chapter in a Collaborative Author Project. We have a spot for you. What will become possible for you when you do this thing?

I opened an all-female publishing house, Red Thread Publishing, devoted to empowering women to find their voice, write their stories, publish their books and change the world. We teach this method that is uniquely feminine and a fresh approach to writing and publishing that breaks out of the old ways that hold us back.

If I had somehow managed to avoid any of my previous struggles, I would not have quite the skill set to do this important work in the world. We do not need to avoid our obstacles or struggles. Rather, I teach a woman how to accelerate her process with ease, so that one obstacle does not make her stuck. Instead, each obstacle teaches her the next thing she needs on her journey, so that she can meet the next obstacle, and the next in quick succession, **learning what she needs to become who she always has been.**

THE STORMS THAT FORGE US

Women come to us with stories in their hearts, a story that must be told. So many of us are often still in the thick of our own storms, drowning in doubt, and the fear and the belief of not enough time, nor enough money. Like willing storm chasers, we get swept up in chaos again and again. Yet our stories still demand to be told.

As hard as it feels to tell your story, as scary as all of that may be, not telling your story will always be heavier and harder than telling it. Instead of just being a publishing company, I'm bringing together all of the pieces of my previous selves: the teacher part, the struggling writer part, and the women's empowerment part. I have woven together all of these skills that I learned and forged in the fire of my own struggle. One of our programs, *The Story Incubator,* teaches a new methodology, that I discovered while writing my first two books, that makes it fun and so much easier to write the deep truths.

Stacy Dyson is a Black American Poet. She has published two collections this summer with Red Thread Books: ***Lovely and Suffering*** and ***Follow Me on This***. Stacy told me, *"Publishing these books saved my life. I've been a poet for over 40 years. But recently I started to wonder if I had any more in me. Putting these books into the world and hearing how they have impacted people has breathed new life into me, and into my work. Now, I know I have a lot more to offer."* It's stories like this that remind me why I do the work that I do. They cultivate my faith.

Kim, a Red Thread Writer, has recently completed our Story Incubator book writing course. She said, *"When I came into it I had no clue, no understanding of how to go about the process. I wanted to tell my story but had no idea how to begin. Now I know that I can write a book! The information was so powerful and it has impacted me. I know where to start now; I have hope, and I know I can always reach out when I get stuck."* We each just need support, and the faith to make it happen.

I always think of this tree. This tree that has half of its leaves falling off. This tree that is going into winter, letting go, and dropping away all of its old, and yet simultaneously, flowers, and young, fresh fragile leaves are unfurling next to old weathered dried leaves. Instead of the deciduous forests of my childhood that drop their leaves and stay barren, for the winter months naked and spindly. These trees. These trees. They're like quantum trees. They're in all phases of life, simultaneously, birth to fullness, aging, withering and death, needing to let go in order to grow.

WHO NEEDS YOUR STORY?

I love the reminder that this tree offers me, the vision that we are always becoming. Like the tree we are always capable of much more than we're aware, and that we believe. I am exactly where I need to be in this moment. But I'm not fooling myself that I will be here like this forever. I've been around the block enough times to know. More storms will come. I'm ready and grateful for them. I have the faith that I will learn exactly what I need to learn from each and that I have the tools to survive and thrive, despite harsh winds.

We write to heal our stories and transform our lives but it goes beyond that. Leslie, another of our Red Thread Writers in the Story Incubator, celebrated her five-year "cancerversary" last month. She doubted her story was worthy of sharing. She said, *"Limiting beliefs and systems were the culprit always holding me back from what I have wanted to write all these years. Now with this process, this is the furthest I have gotten in my book ever. With your direction and guidance, it has made writing a book a lot more fun. Knowing I am part of a community of women really committed to getting their stories out there helps."* By writing your story you can absolutely change the world. Who's ready? (Join our community for free) We are not alone in this journey. We are not alone in this process when we are brave enough, when we are courageous enough to dig into our own struggle, and heal our own stories. When we do this through writing, we can activate quantum impact; transforming ourselves and giving permission to others to do the same.

Where have you been misguided in your own interpretation of who you are and how the world works?

SEEK PROOF

In this chapter, I want to leave you with some ideas about examining your own perception, and to revise your own story about who you are as well as who you can become. I have built an extensive resource vault to support all the emotional and logistical elements of telling your story. One of the tools I offer my women's circles and our community of authors is to *seek proof.* When we come into this place of doubt, recognize the questions that we are asking ourselves. The mind is very efficient. It will answer anything set before it.

I ask "What if you seek proof of all that you *have* accomplished? All that you are capable of? All that is already working for you?"

That day, when I unpacked my life, I wasn't even seeking those things. All I was hoping to do was to declutter those boxes. I discovered something even better there. I discovered a new possibility of myself, a new reality. On the floor that day, I discovered a new perspective that the storms I thought I had been fighting and living through, not only weren't really storms at all, but also that simple shift to choose to look at my experience differently offered possibility for my life rather than disappointment and limitation.

Seek proof of what you want to find and believe.

OWN YOUR STORY

The book is one of the oldest technological societal tools. Yet it is still one of the most powerful to teach, to inspire, to transform. Ideas are the core of who we are. When we allow ourselves to fall victim to limiting beliefs, false ideas still rule to keep us small, to keep us stuck. Owning our own stories and accepting our own darkness gives permission to readers to do the same.

There is very clearly a changing, rising tide. When one woman's perception of herself transforms, she's contributing to the tipping point of the transformation of the consciousness of all of humanity.

We need women's voices in the world. Each individual woman needs to hear her own voice, needs to listen and trust her own inner truth. She needs to discover, like I did, where her stories were constructed on false beliefs.

The mission of Red Thread Publishing, to support women to write and publish their books, allows us to witness women in one of the most potent transformations we can have as adults. It is like hearing the heartbeat of humanity. We get to be the first to hear the newest voices communicating from the depths of their souls. We amplify those voices by bringing their books into the world!

To all the women in the world with a stormy story to tell, I salute you.

THE END

SIERRA MELCHER

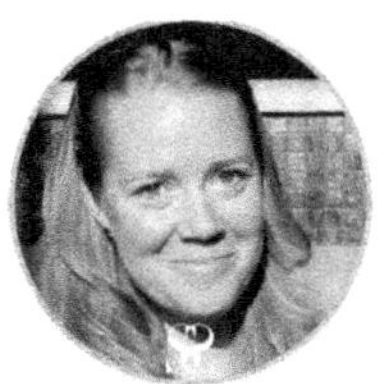

Best-selling author, international speaker & educator, Sierra Melcher is founder of ***Integral Women Institute & Red Thread Publishing LLC.*** Sierra leads an all-female publishing company, supporting women, in every step of the writing & publishing process to empower & elevate the voices of women around the world. Writing & Publishing intentionally accelerates personal, spiritual & professional growth. BECAUSE EVERY STORY MATTERS.

Sierra has a Master's degree in education, has spoken & taught around the world. Originally from the United States, Sierra lives in Medellin, Colombia with her young daughter.

Contact information:
https://linktr.ee/integralwomen

16

SOPHIE'S STORY

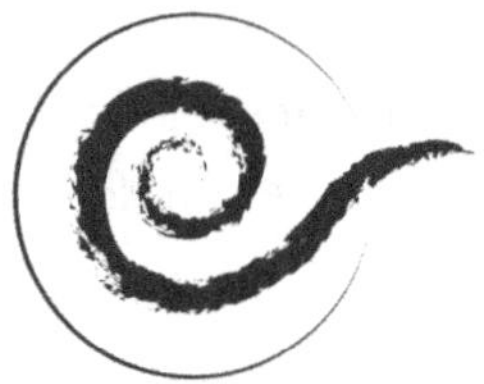

I always knew I was different from other kids. I felt like I was suffocating, trapped in a war zone of a home with a deteriorating alcoholic father, whom I loved very much. I watched him go from a high-flying businessman in chauffeured cars to falling down the alcoholic rabbit hole into a really dark place, and there was nothing I could do to stop him from destroying himself. No amount of love, pleading or threats can stop someone once they've hit the self-destruct button. I got used to doing homework while he was screaming that he wanted to kill himself - it was just another day. I snapped one day, and told him to just do it. Those were my last words to him. That haunted me for a long time. It's impossible to watch the person you're closest to fade away like that, then finally find their body on the way to school one morning. I went to school after finding his body. I have no idea why. But I was picked up in a cop car soon after and taken home to yellow tape and white suits. I went to school the next day. Again, I don't know why. I assume I was on autopilot. But I knew something inside me had changed forever, and I'd never get it (or him) back. Even before that, I felt no connection to the people around me. I didn't function, act, or think like them in any way. I craved freedom, which has become a theme throughout my life

– live alone, achieve financial freedom, work remotely, travel impulsively...

I was diagnosed with numerical dyslexia around this time and was told multiple times I couldn't do this or that. Later I was told that I couldn't study psychology, because 'I wasn't smart enough.' I believed them for a long time. I had horrendous acne as a teenager too, so my self-worth and self-confidence were rock bottom. Perfect prey for men, unfortunately.

I became the class clown because I just wanted to have fun and be free of feeling so deeply unhappy all the time. I was chubby so I got a complex aged 12 and stopped eating, which was noticed, so when I was forced to eat, I started throwing up everything I ate. Then the self-harm started (probably never ended, just manifested in alternative self-destructive behaviors) and the suicide attempts. Because I was from a middle-class white family, no one did a damn thing or asked me what was wrong or tried to intervene. I was first medicated for insomnia, anxiety, and depression aged 11, which sounds crazy, now. I knew for sure by then that I was 'different.' I knew no child my age should feel so desperately unhappy, nor is it normal to be medicated so young. Had people taken the time to figure out why I was so unhappy, maybe things could have been different and life wouldn't have been so difficult.

I had one goal; against all odds, make it to university. I made it, but I should have planned further, because once I made it to Uni, I had zero fucks and no more goals to achieve, so I partied ALL the time.

I finally started fighting back aged 22 and said 'fuck everyone. My life has to mean something so that my father stressing himself to give us the best life while killing himself in the process wasn't in vain.' This has been the driving force behind everything that I do -in addition to the joy of proving everyone wrong and the hunger to create a more than comfortable life for myself.

I retook my science GCSE exam, got an A*, and was accepted into studying medicine, just to prove a point. Yes, I am that petty. I wanted to throw it in everyone's faces that no one has any business telling a child that they can't do something, or that they're not clever enough – what kind of example is that setting?! But on the flip side, their put-downs were the catalyst for change. I started my first business (an entertainment agency) aged twenty-three. It didn't work out and I was down $7000, but it taught me more than any school curriculum or a Business & PR degree ever did.

Fast-forward a few years of abusive, toxic relationships (textbook) including one real prince who pushed me out of a car for 'looking at a guy' and one dating disaster after another... I found myself engaged to someone who tried to cheat on me multiple times (couldn't get that past me, not smart enough), so after 5 years, I ran. I lived in Morocco for 2 years, got engaged to someone I later found out was a conman and hit women, so, I ran again. I met a bunch of army boys from San Diego in a Moroccan nightclub who I flipped a coin with on whether I should move to San Diego or Miami. Miami won, so I ran again, and 5 years later, here I am.

When I arrived in Miami, I had spent all my money on flights and 4 months upfront on an apartment (immigrant tax), so I was sleeping in my South Beach studio on an airbed with no other furniture for 2 months and could barely afford to eat. In that time, I worked on building Brand Branding PR LLC and recruiting social media, branding, marketing, and PR clients. There were times I thought I'd made a mistake relocating to America, and at many times I got anxious and asked myself 'What if this doesn't work? What then? 'There was a time when I lost all three clients on the last day of the month when the end of the year came, as I hadn't made them sign contracts. So yes, that was the first time I ever drank a whole bottle of wine alone and felt defeated. I knew no one when I moved here, so other than befriending promoters, it was isolated.

The thing about entrepreneurism is it's a disease – a good one. Even after the worst of days, you can't help but wake up the next day with a rejuvenated drive to activate your comeback with a vengeance. I had three higher-paid clients within a week. The moral of the story is you can come back from anything no matter how bad you think the situation is. You just need to upgrade your mindset, hit the reset button, and shoot from a different angle.

It's scary relocating. You worry all the time. 'What if?' 'What if?.' When you have no 'real' friends or family nearby, you're in constant fear 'what if my business fails and I can't pay the rent, where will I go? What will happen to me?' When I had three weeks in-between the end of my lease and being able to move into my new apartment, I was lucky enough to have a Michaelangelo in my life who invited me to stay with him, otherwise, who knows...? This is the same guy who offered to look after me after my bike accident even though we hadn't seen each other in a year or so. Real people are hard to find, especially in Miami. I hold them close and consistently think of ways I can repay their kindness once I make my millions.

I eventually moved in with roommates to lessen the financial burden (and isolation), but more importantly, meet decent people instead of the endless fleet of gold digging bottle hoes who swarm the Miami clubs and bars. It's the best decision I ever made. Cat Valiani and Priya Chandel became the sisters I never had, and so the real adventure began...

Soon after, I met who I then thought was the 'love of my life' who wanted to spend every day with me, told everyone we were getting married, then after a few months, completely vanished. I had no idea if he was dead or alive, and the whole experience nearly destroyed me. Eventually we reconnected and three months later, the same thing again, and so the cycle continued, on and off for four to five years until I discovered he had made it clear that he isn't in love with me (and possibly never was). So, while giving me diamonds on my birthday and asking me to have his babies, he was supposedly seeing other girls the whole time. After dealing with so much dating drama in Miami, I'm desensitized at this point. How can you be connected to someone for nearly 5 years, then just push them aside like they're nothing? Welcome to Miami...

At this point I think I have PTSD from dating in Miami. I never experienced such coldness and cruelty in London. I feel like I don't date anymore; I simply foster big kids until they move onto their forever home. I'm not doing this ridiculous dance anymore. I have so much love to give and no outlet for it, so I'd rather put my time and energy into helping kids who really need some love in their lives, and who deserve my time and energy. I saved myself and became my own hero, so now I can do it for others in need by becoming a foster mom in 2022.

Now, I take accountability for the part I played in all of my dysfunctional relationships. The moment you let people back into your life after they fuck you over you write 'doormat' on your forehead in a big, flashing neon sign and set yourself up for heartbreak and toxic attachments.

The rollercoaster ex is super successful now and I couldn't be prouder, but of course, with success and money will come the hoes, which seems to fulfill a need for men here to make them feel like 'the man.' Maybe someday he'll remember that I loved him when he was driving a Volkswagen, way before the boat and the sports car. But in Miami, you tend to regularly be replaced by uneducated, surgically enhanced girls that make a career out of living off men.

I was naive when I moved here, so I needed to learn the lesson not to trust anyone until they earn it, and to observe someone's actions rather than their words – actions tell you everything you need to know about how someone feels about you. The signs are all there, we just choose to ignore our intuition sometimes. Dating experiences in Miami really triggered my self-destructive behaviors. It almost broke me. There were some very, very dark days over the years. I owe my old roommates big time for dealing with my on-off relationship drama. Every. Time.

The positive takeaway is that I met my amazing sister from another mister Precious Totanes-Mcintosh via one of my ultimate dating disasters. Secondly, I no longer allow myself to become so attached to people that I fall apart if and when they leave. That's spiritual and emotional growth right there. Update - six weeks on since writing the original draft for this chapter, I wish him all the happiness in the world but I feel nothing for this dude anymore, and I am happily dating a doctor who knows how to treat a woman, and is crazy enough to want to (currently) marry me. What a pivot. I'd legit given up on ever finding love. Didn't see this one coming...

When you relocate, it's important to build a tribe who supports and loves you unconditionally. I met my 'Nepowman' squad when my now Goddaughter wanted to meet me after watching me take a beer on stage at a blogger event (classic). A few years on, I'm lucky enough to call Jackie, Justin, Mia and Ava Nepola family. When everything goes left, they put me right.

In 2019, I broke my jaw in a bike accident that nearly killed me (drove off a cliff and landed on my face). The irony is, I never wore a helmet while riding motorbikes in Miami, and the one time I wore one, it was smashed to smithereens and saved my life. I couldn't talk, eat or swallow and I looked like a monster. I cried the whole way back to America because I realized I had no one to look after me and that was a moment of suffocating loneliness during the long flight home. I lost a lot of weight after being on a liquid diet for two months. Soon after, I got spotted, scouted, and paid to walk the runways of Miami Swim Week, and just walked in the 2021 shows. I like to see opportunity in everything - when you look at life's challenges this way, you can never fail. I choose not to see obstacles, I see opportunities. Pivot and play.

Moving into my own condo in 2021 was the best decision I made in a long time. I'm sound sensitive and need alone time, so I have been in my element plotting and creating. I became a contributing writer to Forbes and Entrepreneur, won multiple business awards, became a best-selling author, and have two patented brands coming out in 2022.

The biggest lessons I learned in 2021 is that you can be successful, financially independent, and a bikini model and the majority of men still won't give a shit, nor see or understand your worth; they'd rather be around women who 'need' them financially because it feeds their ego and they don't have to make any effort to keep these girls. Second, once you reach a certain level of success, many of your friends won't support you anymore; your greatness makes them uncomfortable. So, we have to learn to clap for our damn selves and become the hero of our own stories. And thirdly, men say they want an attractive, successful, and intelligent woman, but most of them don't; it challenges them to step up and makes them feel inferior. Shut that shit down and send them on their merry way to settle down with a gold digging hoe who will lie, cheat and steal. In a month or two, they always realize their mistake and try to come back... don't open the door to them. Karma is a bitch. What can a man who judges his desirability and worth to women based on his net worth offer a woman who has her own empire? Nothing. So, they run away with their tail between their legs and a bruised ego to 'save' the nearest damsel in distress to validate their narcissism.

This is why it's SO important to work on liking your own company and make moves to build belief in yourself to ensure you don't let these mother fuckers break you. The moment you stop measuring your self-worth on how others treat you is the point where you evolve, elevate your life, and become UNFUCKWITHABLE.

The norm when you win big is to go out and celebrate with friends. When I made two huge life-changing wins in one week, I was really upset by the lack of interest or support from friends who knew how much it means to me to 'make it', and how hard I sacrificed and hustled to achieve this milestone. Then, I caught myself. Why put that kind of power into the hands of others? It was me that won. No one else. So, I upgraded the celebration process to simply take time out, give thanks, sit on my balcony looking over the water reminiscing about everything I went through to get to where I am and just radiate gratitude. I may even book a trip or organize something fun I've wanted to do for ages, or buy myself something significant.

In summary, there is opportunity in everything. You can break any negative cycle when you CHOOSE to. You can always find your tribe wherever you are in the world. We can bounce back no matter how bad it is. And I have (had) really bad taste in men.

I haven't allowed myself to let go of my former acceptance of being alone forever yet. My behavior at times pushes people away, and I've accepted that I'm too much for most people. Accepting yourself for who you are is the key to inner peace. Know that the right people will love you no matter how alone you may feel now, and you'll know it in your soul when you find your person - or when they find you. Nothing you do can push your real ones away, no matter how fucked up you're told your demeanor can be at times.

Keeping the 'fire in your belly' alive, persevering towards your goals despite dodging constant curveballs from the universe, and remembering there is always a solution is how you weather the storms of life and become STORMBORN. To be continued...

SOPHIE BOWMAN

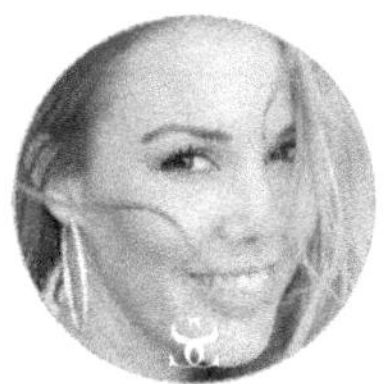

Founder of convertyourfollowers.com, award-winning Forbes-published entrepreneur & best-selling author.

https://www.instagram.com/sophiecbowman/
https://convertyourfollowers.com/

17

THE WARRIOR'S PATH

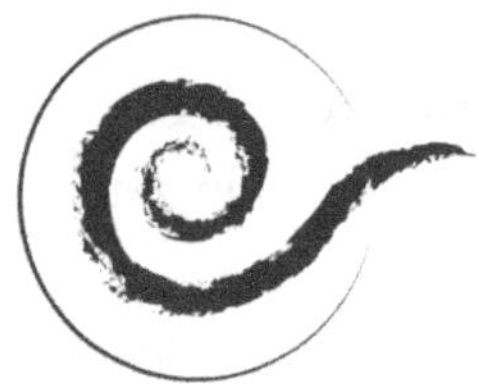

"The world breaks everyone and afterward many are strong in the broken places."
Ernest Hemingway

It was all so many years ago.

And still such feelings arise! Writing this chapter has evoked and re-awakened the sleeping giant of pain, so more buried layers can come up for healing. That is how healing works - layer after layer reveals to allow more healing.

WARRIORS TRAIN

Warriors are trained by life, shaped by the elemental forces, forged from courage and discipline, and deepened through practice.

For me, you cannot be a warrior without training. That is the path, testing one's bravery, courage, wisdom, determination, discipline, grace, self-awareness, and compassion for self. There is much to learn, not just sword work and steps. It's life practice.

To become a warrior, you must commit to do the training. To teach people about warrior training you need to humbly accept your path, and go through your own cycles of learning, developing trust in the process.

So I share my stories of how I have learned to stand, ground, centre and find myself in the storm. A kind Scottish man once told me, in my mid thirties, as my marriage of fifteen years fell apart and my career reached a savage peak of demanding pressure, that his grandmother had told him – "Billy boy, when you are in a big storm and you cannot find your way ... stand still."

I have dwelt upon this quote much in the years since – don't run around in the dark, don't act in blindness ... you might fall over a cliff in a huge mist of storm and rain. No, when you are lost - be still. Wait for the clouds to clear. They will.

This knowing when to move and when to be still is key in the martial arts training I practice, known as Aikido. I have practiced Aikido on the mat and off the mat for many years. My deepest love is to use Aikido off the mat, which means in my daily life.

Harnessing energy coming towards you, and sending it back where it came, is a part of martial arts training. As are practices of blending, centering and developing harmony. Such mighty principles are seen on the mat, and take practice! The biggest power we have is using energy, insight and intention with ourselves.

> *"Knowing others is wisdom. Knowing self is enlightenment."*
>
> *Lao Tzu*
>
> *"Your spirit is your true shield."*
>
> *Morihei Ueshiba, (O Sensei), founder of Aikido.*

The black belt is a sign of intense and long training.

The Jedi are trained by Yoda.

Aikido is its own Samurai training.

The student respects the teacher who assists them in their development. And, of course, the ultimate teacher is life.

The teachers and supportive ones appear ... as we need them!

Here are my two biggest storms of testing ...

THE COLLAPSE OF EVERYTHING

I am 34 years old. My heart has split, as my beloved Grandmother has just died. My protector, soul mother, axis. And now my marriage collapses in the same year. 34 was the most heart-wrenching time of my life.

Oddly in recent days - while writing this chapter - my daily diaries from that time synchronistically appeared. So I have read them and relived the agonizing loss and confusion. Turmoil indeed.

I was just 17 when we talked all night and he kissed me passionately on the steps.

Already friends, this deep place of us was like home, and just before I turned 20 we married, three years later to the day. We were different but close. Opposites attracted. We were spiritually aligned.

All aspects of our life were great and fulfilling, until just the end period of our 17 years together. Our friends wished plaintively they had a relationship as good as ours.

Jump ahead 14 years from our wedding day ... we were both busy in huge careers, losing each other in different timetables and horrendous work pressures, turning inwards just to survive! We took different exploratory turns in our life journey. Unthinkable that after 17 years that we would end ... but we did.

Sorrow ... as I started the questioning ... definitely wondering who else I could become. And how to evolve. But he finished it, decisively.

And never opened the door again, despite six months of marriage counselling.

We made love one mind-blowing passionate last time. Break-up sex I think. And it was over.

Neither of us were unfaithful, it was a shared train track that had forked into two different tracks now. We no longer shared and we had our own ideas of what we wanted. He met his next wife quickly, as men often do.

She was cruel as hell to me. It's hard enough when couples split up, worse in a way when the relationship has been mightily good.

But such cruelty she threw at me! Shattered and forlorn without him, I had to accept they had now begun, but I missed him still. There was much to unravel yet we spoke little once separated. I found it hellish, missing my life companion.

Though she never met me, his new partner left cruel messages on my mobile, sent horrible embarrassing messages to my shared work email and insulted me with taunts and cruel comparisons.

Unnecessary injury. He and I had split before they met.

They had (it seemed from afar, and he did confirm) a bumpy time in the first years.

It was bad enough the utter life change of 17 years together just disappearing ... but now seared with the blow torch of her cruel vicious taunting .... I fell to pieces.

She and I were strangers but somehow she thought it ok to contact me from America and leave hurtful messages for me. It broke my heart what she said that he said about me too. Nothing made sense of the life we had shared. I tried tranquilizers for a month. Not for me! So I danced four nights a week at Sydney Dance company, sweating and whirling out pain.

Brief bragging phone message taunted cruelly and deepened the scar -

Dig the knife in, why don't you? Where do women get such cruelty towards other women? She had never met me but kicked me when I was down. Others have said I must have been so alive in his psyche, she must have had insecurities, but the level of cruelty she poured on me from across the globe shocked me.

Such sadness arose - that this was who he chose as a worthy replacement wife. She is a trauma "expert" apparently. Well good on her for creating some for me! Forgiving this woman has been harder than releasing the man I had known and loved all those years. I forgave, as best I could, her need to injure as part of her process.

Healing has so many layers, I know, and just writing about this era has shown me more layers of healing, surfacing to heal. Wounds leave scar tissue and I have mine. I have been shocked to find such tenderness in the scars. They took a long time to heal back then.

So there I was - 35 years old - alone in our lovely big house.

Now divorced.

Achingly missing my life companion.

Working long hours setting up my new corporate communication agency.

Confused in solo identity, having been in a couple my whole adult life.

Dating and finding new passions, mistakes and loves.

Missing my old life (so good until we lost each other).

Doing psychotherapy and learning bio-energetics, Reich, Jung and the pioneers of psychology.

Investigating so many types of body therapies and deep release work, mindfulness trainings and healing modalities. This time built me anew.

I learnt to be alone. I bought a bush block once we sold the house, and learnt to be safe in my own company on the land, in deep nature.

I learnt to dance more freely, my own dance therapy of sorts, to release the pain. Yes I learnt to dance in the rain, literally and metaphorically.

My business thrived, I grew in my potency.

Eventually, I could be on my land, alone in the bush land and unafraid. Travel alone internationally.

I became my own warrior.

My own true love.

Shattered open by cataclysmic loss and change, slowly I built a new life, with a new sense of self. New chapters began.

DANCE WITH DYING

The car spun badly, out of control.

I thought I was going to die.

I didn't ...

But my spirit shot up and over the top of the car, out of my body.

I lost control twice, regained in the flash of swerving, knowing to steer into the skid, but not brake too hard or I would spin even more.

The third time I lost it. The smash was enormous as we collided, on a quiet road in the Australian bush.

Images of the World Trade Towers collapsing crumbled around me in a swirl of gum trees and gravel.

At that moment, I softened.

Feeling the impact of a head-on collision absorb into my bones,

I let my tight adrenal grasping of the steering wheel soften.

"This is it", I thought.

Miraculously I survived, but I was a changed woman. That flash didn't come – life before my eyes – but I did truly think this was my ending. I collapsed in shock on the ground once I got out of the car, dazed and shattered, on the curving bush road that fateful Spring evening.

Many aspects of my life changed after that massive head-on collision car crash, at age 41. Firstly, I was in agonising guilt for a long while, as it was my car that had spun on the loose gravel roadwork surface. I was in a big car with airbags, unlike the badly injured woman, whose car I had collided with, on a road surface that felt like marbles.

Next followed a court case funded by loans and financial setbacks, to pay a barrister and road traffic expert to explain what happened.

A year of fear, anxiety, worry.

Most importantly in this upheaval, facing serious charges, I learnt about letting in love ... the care of others, the support of friends, the feeling of knowing it was not my time yet. And learnt to use dance as my primary therapy to heal the body and psyche trauma of such a big crash.

I had to rebuild my life in a new way - refinance, move house, close my communications agency and move out of Sydney to live in the country .... all to heal my altered nervous system. My psyche craved quiet and my need to balance my life was immense.

Before the crash, life was frantically busy. 12-15 hour working days, endless travel, weekend work. Now, post the crash, I sat stunned in the sun for a week, my energy feeling fragile and fine shatter lines through me, like a Japanese crazed Raku pottery piece, feeling astonished for being alive at all.

Everything was poignantly crisp. In focus. Astonishingly beautiful.

Over the ensuing months the crash brought mild whiplash (no fun), massive learning about chiropractors and energy healing, and going deeper in discovering for myself the healing power of dance.

I danced each night in my wee little south coast beach cottage.

Unravelling, decompressing, being with the shock, the endless flashbacks that stopped me sleeping, releasing the body trauma packed inside. Without knowing it, I was using all the training I had so far in my long journey over a decade to become a qualified dance movement therapist.

I used everything I had learnt (and experimented too), to heal my fractured body, psyche and energy systems. It was a revelation.

Dance is my bedrock place of expression - for processing life, for releasing energy, for reviewing my experiences, for allowing the moving body to show me the truth of my desires and needs. My dance journey had begun at age four, with beloved classical ballet and extended later to jazz, contemporary and later still to improvised and ecstatic dance meditation. Finding dance as the primary therapy was its own journey, and this car crash was a huge lesson and deepening for me.

There have been many trials since, but I always turn to dance to find my own resilience in expressing grief and losses, integrating and processing them, transforming them into the gold of learning and healing.

The energy of that huge car crash shook me to my cells. The movement work I explored as part of my healing became a deepening gold vein that still exists in my therapeutic work today. The whole experience took me deeper in understanding trauma, healing, compassion and using movement, witnessing and presence to rebuild one's life.

TRANSFORMATION IS INTENSE

I now love wildness.

I am fine with aloneness.

I love storms.

I revel in the power of nature.

I live where winds roar and the sea pounds with passion.

I have transformed the upheaval of the storms in my life.

Transformation is no gentle process but one of dissolution, upheaval, chaos and surrender. These days an image of a Phoenix image sits above my mantelpiece in swirling reds and golds ... reminding me daily that life will lead to transformation, anchoring my warrior spirit in the possible movements of change.

Here is a poem I wrote recently to express the intensity of transformation:

PHOENIX May 2021

In a fluttering storm
Of ferocious feathery ascent,
Scrambling from black ashes,
Mystery takes form,
As this new bird, surprisingly, rises.

Confused, I watch,
As all that was

(Poof) disappears
In ashen dust,
And the ugly newness
Of unknown strange differentness,
Unsteadily flaps me.

Screeches of a new potent beginning,
No gentle thing,
But raging elevation
From the fire of transformation.

Freed from a burning death -
Phoenix rises.
Defiant.
Exhilarant.
New.
Trans
Formed.

Intensity and drama enravel the Phoenix as it rises from the ashes, now a new creation. Just like the chrysalis holds the caterpillar as it fully dissolves its form to re-organise totally into new form as a butterfly, so a new form of life and being comes. The mighty experiences of challenge, trials and upheaval bring us to the cliff or through the storm or the fire to an ending of our known landscapes ... where our new world of transformation can occur.

I revel in my warrior Celtic and Viking roots. I am not scared of storms.

I have been in huge storms where gum trees split in half and windows smashed inwards. I have been in the firestorm winds of the recent cataclysmic Australian bushfires with smoke and ash and heat all around.

I have swirled in a collision of car metal glass. I have lost my dearest and held the hands of death.

And all this prepared me for my career, helping others to transform their lives. Whether doing executive leadership coaching, private counselling, couples work, life transitions, dance therapy with dementia patients or mental health carers, or assisting those seeking to explore moving their challenges and lives - I lean fully into what I learnt in these primary experiences of devastation and transformation in my own life.

Each of us has testing or storms in our lifetime. I am sure of this, after 20 years sitting in intimate sharing as an executive coach and therapist. I own my storms and know them as my territory of learning.

I have learnt to trust the body's wisdom, expression and capacity for healing; the power of movement; the power of the breath to release and change; the intimacy of vulnerability; the potency of words and touch; and the conversational learning possible in the meeting of true presence, compassion and clear mind in a held environment.

I love how my work is the territory of learning that arose from my lessons in my storms. Does my life feel like I overcame it all? No. It's moving.

It's a work in progress. We re-gather as the next level of tests and training continue.

Life is vibrancy, like a fire, a refining, a proving, a process. An alchemy that continues on. The provings keep coming. But arising from the heat is joy, continual learning and sharing, love and intimacy, rebuilding and deepening connection, expansive peace and vulnerable surrender.

Beloved reader - stay true to your spirit.

You are a warrior of wisdom.

Sovereign in your choices.

I will keep helping leaders create their intentions, ignite their vision, inhabit their bodies, their potential and their magnificence, living their leadership from spiritual and emotional intelligence.

It's awesome to know one's capacity. I have learnt not to abandon myself in tornadoes of work challenges, or the storms of relationship trials. You keep humble when you know how much has conspired to help you survive and thrive.

If you are looking for your soul business I can help you envision it.

If you know you need to transition to a new life, it is my joy to help.

If you want to open up your potential, or be a better leader of your life or your business, I can journey alongside and show you how.

A number of times I have wobbled - career or heartbreak again subsuming my life. I get off-centre yes. But I trust my inner warrior - and while people and situations can affect me - the art and practice is to continually return back to my centre and practice once again.

These days need warriors, Phoenix-like, trained in wisdom, balanced in their energies, fearless, self-sovereign, authentic, clear thinking and committed with courage and presence to live one's values.

In the turmoil currently on Earth we need to remember that we are connected through love, and our light is the expression of infinite love.

So dear reader, be brave now. In order to rise in your own life, like a Phoenix in the fires of transformation, practice like a warrior. Lead your life with wisdom.

I encourage you to walk with courage the deep path of transformation to your highest magnificent self.

VIRGINIA SADA YORK

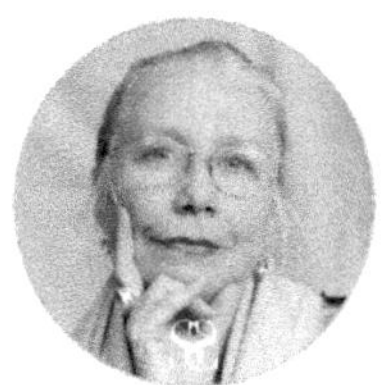

Virginia Sada York, founder of Your World Within, works with transformation and movement, as executive leadership coach, facilitator and dance movement therapist. Her work catalyses movement and growth in CEOs, start-ups, team leaders and individuals, using artistry and warrior practices of leadership to radiate success.

In her vibrant global coaching practice and online programs, Virginia ignites transformation, combining whole body awareness, purpose, vision, courage and wisdom, integrating feminine and masculine energies, practising work/home life balance, and awakening each person to their authentic talents and potency.

Virginia helps leaders utilise all of themselves - mind, body, spirit - using body energetics, clearing and movement practices, pragmatically combined with business strategy and visionary creativity to unleash the alchemy of change.

Virginia is also CEO of Alchemy Publishing, which activates transformation for conscious business, sharing stories from potent women about their work creating new paradigms of healing, community and learning in the world.

Contact information: https://linktr.ee/virginiasadayork

18

YVONNE'S STORY

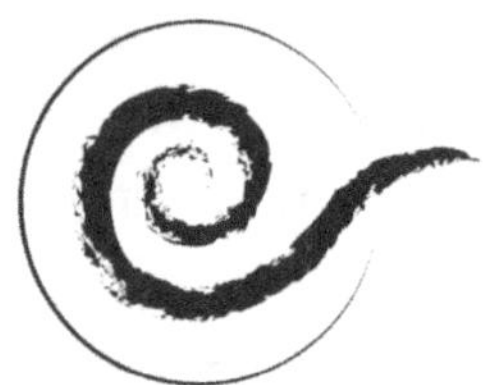

How many of you know that there comes a point in life when certain things get in the way of you fulfilling your dreams and goals? Raise your hands please.

Thank you.

Ladies and gentlemen, I want you to think about your goals and dreams. And as you think about them right now, here is something I want to say to you: you are going to face some challenges, you are going to run into some difficulties.

There are some things that are going to happen to you and take you unaware.

And I want you to write this down: 'YES' What will happen is that life can knock you down silly.

And you begin to operate in fear, doubt and disorientation.

I am talking to you from a place I lived for a very long time.

A place I was put under fear, self-doubt and confusion.

STORMBORN is a masterpiece filled with captivating life stories that will leave you with great lessons of courage, hope, self-confidence and support as you navigate the uneven waters of life.

This masterpiece confirms my conviction that everything that happens to you, happens for you.

Life as it is, is full of a mixture of adventures.

It is our attitude towards it that determines which way we go.

I am 11 year old.

Sitting in the kitchen surrounded by my brothers, grandmother and my father.

My father in anger tells my grandmother he wants me to get married to a man of his choice.

Dead silence filled the kitchen.

My father said again to my grandmother "do you hear what I am telling you?

More dead silence and fear fills the kitchen.

Reflecting over the years, my grandmother explains to my father how disappointed she is in the way my mother and her children are being abused.

She tells my father that my granddaughter is too young to get married.

I would like her to be educated like your legal older girls as well.

What followed this conversation almost left my grandmother dead if my brother had not sneaked out to summon an elderly neighbor.

My father never wanted me or loved me as his child unless I did what he wanted me to do.

He arranges for me to marry a man I don't know nor love.

He tells me "Mundih, unless you do what I ask you to do, you will never amount to anything."

Unless you marry, you will sleep in the bush among animals.

It's important to know the origin of my father's hatred, abuse and rejection of me.

My mother was married at age 16.

Within two years, she gave birth to twin girls.

Shortly after, her husband was killed by my biological father.

Her home was demolished and all her husband's property seized.

She was rendered homeless while the twins were still breastfeeding.

My father raped my mom in the filthiest of places.

She got pregnant with me.

She was forced to live in my father's compound among his wives and children, some of whom were around my mother's age.

Ladies and gentlemen, I am a positive by-product of rape.

When I was three years old, my father gave me away despite the cries and pleads of my mother.

I embark on a foster care journey.

This same journey was the beginning of my journey to freedom.

In these homes, I was abused as well.

The only difference was that I slept inside, ate sometimes and I was sent to school.

At 11 after primary school, my father ordered that I be sent home.

My arrival at the village was the beginning of my father forcing me into marriage.

My mother ended up with 9 kids of her own.

All of us were abused and rejected.

It was hard.

I contemplated suicide and actually prayed to God to take my mother and her children or at least end my life.

When my grandmother left my father's compound, at midnight my father sent me out of the house.

I groped my way around the village to a neighbor's house.

With a lighted bush lamp, the neighbor took me across the river to my grandmother.

My father found out and threatened my grandmother and all the villagers to never take me in.

He was a terror to the village.

All the villagers were afraid to take me in.

Every midnight my father would send me out of the home.

I started sleeping in the bush as no one would take me in.

Hunger, fear, and dirt infested me.

On their way to the farm early in the morning, the village women would stealthily and kindly drop food on plantain leaves for me to eat in the bush.

I wandered around during the day to find palm kennels and fruits to eat if the village women did not bring me food.

I was terrified.

I was lonely, fearful and I cried everyday hoping I would die.

I felt treated unfairly as I watched other kids going to school.

Then one day, one elderly neighbor asked to send me away to the city to be a housekeeper since I was unwanted.

My father said take her, I don't care.

About a year as a housekeeper, my father again ordered that I'd be sent home to get married.

I am 12 years old now.

Back in the village,

Though unhappy, I was glad I was back in the village.

My main concern now was to protect my mother and my siblings as they could not speak for themselves, especially my mom who was going through a lot in the hands of my father.

With the teachings and blessings of my grandmother, I made the decision to work hard and build my mom a home and make her happy like other moms.

One day I asked my mom if we could run away from my father's compound to a distant land for refuge.

She could not give me a definite answer.

Her answer was in her sobs as she raised her hands to God in prayer.

She tells me "My daughter, the horse that does not have a tail, it is only God who sends its flies away".

At this point, I began to search my soul and ask a series of questions.

Why my mother and her children?

Why me?

At this point, I felt really rejected.

I felt like an outcast.

I felt like I would never amount to anything.

The bitterness against my father grew.

One day, my father loaded a gun to go and shoot my mother.

God had long ago removed my mother from our one bedroom home to safety.

At this point I began to question my existence.

I asked myself if I would ever get out of this abusive situation.

I became even more bitter.

I hated my father so much so that I began to isolate myself.

I became too quiet.

I started believing in the lies my father told me.

That I would never amount to anything unless I did what he asked me to do.

This took a toll on my mother and my siblings who were very afraid of what my father is capable of doing.

One of my brothers cried for two days without eating.

Everything at this point weighed my mom down.

She developed different health issues and the worst one was stomach ache and forgetfulness.

With no one to protect us, I told myself that I deserve better for me, my mom and my siblings.

I assured my mom and siblings that I would stay strong and work hard for all of us.

I felt I deserved a better life and not just to please my father.

I decided that I wanted to go to school to improve my life.

My mom was unable to pay my way to school.

I decided to do farming and selling vegetables and other small businesses.

Next year I got enrolled in secondary school.

This was exciting.

I admired the educated people so much.

After secondary school, I asked my mother to enroll me in High School.

Seeing how determined I was, my mother agreed to sponsor me further with the help of my grandmother.

This reminded me of the teachings of my grandmother who said "There has not been any truly happy and successful person with an easy past".

And she said "Without any pain, there will be no gain in life".

"You are a child of the Highest God, and no weapon fashioned against you shall prosper".

And I remembered the old African proverb that she always reminded us of, "If there is no enemy within, the enemy outside can do us no harm".

I graduated from High school with flying colors.

Now I decided that I will go to university.

My mom became very skeptical.

She explained to me that "My daughter, I really want you to be highly educated because I never went to school".

But our problems might get worse because you will become the first female child of this village to attend higher education.

At this point, all I wanted was to better my life and that of my mom and siblings.

Behold, the universe was on my side.

All the parents of this village came together in kind and cash and decided to send me to university.

You know there is the saying that "One good turn deserves another and even better".

During vacation I always spent it in the village, reading, writing, doing community work, helping to cook for the old and the young, teaching Sunday school and writing letters and mailing them to the parents of the village.

I became the village courier.

This paid off as I got enrolled.

I graduated and became the very first female child in the village for more than ten years with a bachelor's degree.

It was and is still a big deal to me.

I am so grateful.

I have come to realize that in life if you don't fight for what you want, what you don't want will automatically kick in for you.

I had to fight for my life, that of my mom and siblings through hard work and education.

Throughout my education, I did farming and marketing to support my family with education and to learn trades.

Life is hard, but I have learned that when life is hard, play it hard with determination and consistency.

The one who is determined to win is the one who makes breakthroughs.

I was determined to win and to be the first one to eliminate poverty, homelessness, hunger, rejection, abuse, fear and squalor in my family.

The God of the universe paved the way for me even when I did not see a way.

One time I went to watch TV from the only TV owner in the village.

It talked about freedom and opportunities in America.

Without knowing America, I became so obsessed about coming to America that I almost went insane.

My grandmother prayed and told me that the big bird flying in the sky will take me to America.

I was happy.

Still in search of love and acceptance, I got married to a man I loved and he took me to the United States.

The moment we arrived in the US, the relationship became very abusive. I ended up in the shelter for battered women.

This was the moment of reality for me.

I felt like this was another version of my father.

I felt like I would never be loved and accepted, I will never amount to anything like my father had labelled me with.

Still determined to make life better for me, I worked hard and enrolled in school.

I did some side businesses and worked at the same time.

After some years, I decided to marry again just to feel accepted and loved.

This once again was another bad choice.

Within one year, he became exploitative and physically abusive.

I ended up with a second divorce.

I was left alone, lost and very down, and with my son to take care of alone.

This was the moment of truth for me.

The paradigms in my head told me I am worthless, you will never amount to anything.

I felt like I made the wrong choices just to please somebody else.

It was like I was at the end of a cul de sac.

All of these took a toll on my mother and my brothers as well because they looked up to me.

I learned that where there is a will, there is a way. And sometimes when things begin to shake in our lives, it is actually God that is doing the shaking in order to thrust us to a better destination. I was determined to conquer, reign, and build an Empire of my own.

As I struggled, there was something in me that said I will overcome all my difficulties.

I got enrolled into a university and at the same time working.

I graduated and secured a job.

I did gardening and garage sales to augment my income.

Then all of a sudden, my mentor grandmother passed.

My 2 brothers also passed leaving behind little angels.

All together one biological and nine adopted children, including my sick mother rested on my shoulders.

I invited my mom.. She got to the States in a very unsteady condition.

She got diagnosed with a stomach aneurysm and was ordered for immediate surgery or else she would die.

I had to come up with a big down payment as she did not have insurance.

I was in a state of confusion.

I began a ritual of gratefulness in all situations and I took pride in the fact that I am still standing. I began to believe that out of my rocky journey comes purpose, hope and a lesson for someone who is waiting to be uplifted.

I thought about how far I have come in life. I came to the conclusion that God has a Divine appointment and purpose for my life. I thought about this little girl who has the same resemblance as my late little sister who died of abuse at the age of 8. This little girl like me was going through abuse and rejection like me. This little girl also died at age 7. My mother tried adopting her and her father refused. This haunted me for a long time and I decided that I will stand up to speak and advocate for the abused, rejected, the poor, hungry, abandoned, the sick and those pushed to the backwaters of life for no fault of their own. I began to journal everyday. My journals were seized, burnt or thrown away. My grandmother performed a traditional ritual and buried my hopes and dreams in a plastic bag.

In the midst of all of these, I cried out to God for help.

All of a sudden one Sunday as I was seated at my job in tears, a flash of light went through my mind. A voice like that of my grandmother said to me “Stand up and wipe your tears, things are getting better for you, be a mantle”.

I took the phone out of my pocket and started googling seminars.

I found two and I got enrolled.

This is how I started my journey of personal growth and development.

I tried Mary K, Avon and the real estate business and failed.

Then my breakthrough came. A friend invited me to join a speaker and coach training.

I took a leap of faith and I joined.

I even took a bigger leap of faith and invested money that I borrowed from my son. I am now treading the great waters of my destiny and abundance. And I am so grateful to and for my son.

Though afraid because of my past failures, I decided to put my son's money at risk. I have learned that Life is full of risk even when you are eating. So I took it and had the strong belief that I will succeed this time by consistently taking daily actions.

My life took a different turn entirely.

Now I feel a kind of unexplainable spirit of excitement within me every day. I am now a co-author of two books. Amazing.

I am now sharing my knowledge and skills to impact others.

I am now a happy, healthy, wealthy, and passionate woman ready to take the world by storm!

I see the benefits of persistence, self-love, belief and gratitude.

I am indeed a bundle of goodness and kindness to the world put together by my creator to create for others.

What are you doing with the lighted candle the Creator of the universe has given you?

If you can dream it, you can do it. Live, love, build, create and let others do the same with you.

No matter my past, success is part of my DNA. Life is a continuous fight to conquer new territories for the one who is able to. Use your inner gifts to build Monuments in places where STARS are born out of scars.

Be grateful for your adversities. Adversities are blessings in disguise and precious gifts to build, to grow and to conquer.

Redefine, recreate and rewrite your story with a new voice, a new dance and a clean chapter for your life.

Don’t take things personally, it's life.

Always remember where you have been, where you come from and where you are going. Get a road map for your life and help others do better.

Live full and die empty.

Life is sweet and bitter, but it is more sweet than bitter. It is a beautiful blend. Enjoy it.

STORMBORN is an amazing masterpiece filled with lessons and fun discussions that uplifts you and gives you hope to live a better life. I am grateful.

I am a STAR born out of Scars.

If I can do it, so can you.

Thank you.

YVONNE MUNDIH MBUUH

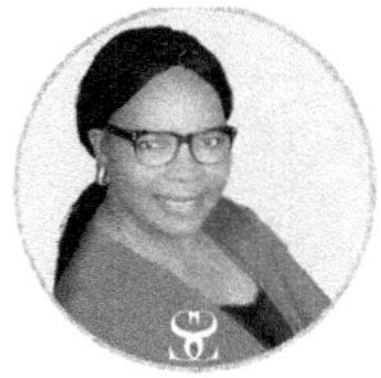

Yvonne is a positive by-product of rape, rejection and abuse.

Living life with passion and purpose are lessons Yvonne learned which have helped her to tread the troubled waters of life, and to become a powerful, determined, unstoppable woman prepared to rewrite a new chapter in her story.

At age 11, Yvonne was forced into marriage against her will. Her refusal plunged her into terrible abusive situations.

Through it all, she placed her trust in God, her mother, and grandmother, and she was determined to conquer and help others.

Her passion to serve helped heal her scars and gave her the strength to help others.

She graduated from The Les Brown Power Voice academy in 2021 and is speaking on platforms across the world sharing her unique story to help victims of domestic abuse.

She is a co-author of two books: 'STORMBORN" and "Hear Her Roar."

https://www.facebook.com/yvonne.mbuuh

https://www.instagram.com/yvonnembuuh/

https://www.linkedin.com/in/yvonne-mundih-mbuuh-369154186

http://tiktok.com/@buildinghopesndreams

https://twitter.com/buildinghopesn1?s=09

https://youtube.com/channel/UCatcjZJe-uqgS-AGZtoFxMQ

https://www.bhdg.org/

WITH GRATITUDE

I would like to extend a big thank you to everyone of our authors who dared to share their stories in this empowering book. This is how you create a legacy and change the world!

In addition to my fantastic authors, I have some special persons that I would like to extend an extra big thank you to, for enabling me to keep the space needed for this book to reach the stars:

- **Mattias Marklund** for his love, support and encouragement.
- **Charlotte Delphi Björndotter** for her proofreading talent.
- **Mira Hilaria Mård** for stepping in when things needed to be organized.
- **The Team at Business Bravery** for seeing our vision and helping us reach our goals and beyond.
- **Stephanie Wicker** at **Muse Designs**, for her amazing creative gifts where she breathes life into my inner images.
- **Colleen Reagan Noon,** for her patience, guidance and support.

With love, *Eleonor Amora*

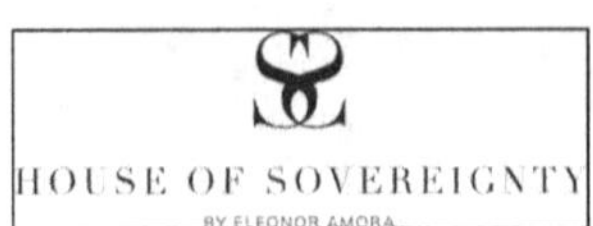
HOUSE OF SOVEREIGNTY
BY ELEONOR AMORA

DISCLAIMER

All similarities with real events or people, living or dead, are just coincidences. All chapters should be seen as fictional.

All writers only stand for their own text in their own chapter and have no responsibility for other individual authors in the book.

www.ingramcontent.com/pod-product-compliance
Lightning Source LLC
LaVergne TN
LVHW010059170826
845678LV00012B/2181

* 9 7 8 9 1 5 1 9 9 2 0 9 9 *